STAND TALL

A Journey from Boy to Man to Master

Andy Dickinson

Praise for Stand Tall

"An inspiring read written by a true warrior. Andy faces the challenges in life with courage."

Peter FitzSimons – Journalist, Bestselling author and Speaker

"A vivid and absorbing story of an exciting fighting life."

Mark Dapin – Award winning author and Journalist

"Andrew, firstly I would like to say how brave you are. Not only about sharing your disease, but also about sharing your life. It is an effortless read and swims off the pages at you. It also chronicles the trials and tribulations of a warrior who refuses to give over control to an unseen foe. I knew you as a warrior and a pathfinder when my children took classes at the Balmain PCYC, and I feel that the Parkinson's disease is yet another belt you must conquer. The warmth and ownership of the story allows us to really see your world and feel your pain, and it also allows us to find out about the man behind the black belt.

It reminds me of a couple of things. God never gives you a dream that matches your budget. He doesn't check your bank account. He checks your faith. Great things never came from the comfort zone. If you want to achieve greatness, stop asking for permission.

It was a pleasure reading this my friend. May the force be with you."

Jay Laga'aia – Actor, Singer, Writer, Early Childhood Educator and father of 8

"Although I have only known Andy for two years now after meeting through our common bond of Parkinson's, his 'good bloke' attitude was immediately noticed. Andy is a fighter in many ways that run far deeper than throwing punches. His passion for improving people's lives through teaching Japanese Ju Jitsu allows him to live out his purpose whilst making a fantastic difference to the people under his guidance.

We are still early on life's journey, and I really look forward to many fun years ahead with Andy leading the way as he has done throughout his life so far."

Clyde Campbell – Founder of the Shake It Up Foundation

"When I walked into my first Taeko class with Andy 18 years ago, the energy was palpable. Andy embodied an attitude and approach to life that made you think anything was possible. Since then, I've seen him grow his business, mentor students and touch the lives of many. His story helps you realise you can deal with whatever the world throws at you. And that is truly inspirational."

Valerie Khoo – Founder and CEO of the Australian Writers' Centre

"It has been my great pleasure to have known Andy since the end of 2011. During that time he has trained with me in Eastern philosophy and meditation, particularly from the yoga-tantra tradition. This training focuses on the development of mental and spiritual power. The aim of the teaching is to become a spiritual warrior – one who can conquer their internal demons, and who can cultivate inner peace and equanimity while facing loss as well as gain and the slaps and blows of life. Andy has shown himself to be a true spiritual warrior, bringing his martial arts spirit into the inner arena where he has won many bouts (and lost a couple too), and of course has many more bouts to face in the future. It has been a privilege to teach Andy over these years and I know he will be a credit to the yoga-tantra tradition as he has been to his martial arts training."

Dr Swami Shankardev Saraswati – www.bigshakti.com

"A fascinating insight into the rugged life of a bouncer from a wise insightful human. Andy is a great man with immense integrity and honour. If there is anyone who can take on the challenge of Parkinson's disease it is Andy."

Tom Cronin – Founder of The Stillness Project

Published by Andrew Dickinson
www.andydickinson.com.au
The moral right of the author has been asserted.

For quantity sales or media enquiries, please contact the publisher at the website address above.

Cataloguing-in-Publication entry is available from the National Library of Australia.

ISBN: 978-0-6484350-0-6 (paperback)
          978-0-6484350-1-3 (ebook)

Editing by Valerie Khoo
Proofreading by Bill Harper
Cover Design by Miladinka Milic
Formatting by Author Secret
Publishing Consultant Linda Diggle

For my Liz

Contents

I love Australia and love the bush. Aussies are renowned for their fighting spirit. In all the wars they have been deeply respected for their bravery and mateship. I took the ideal of 'having a go' and 'giving it my best shot', two great Australian phrases, with me around the world on my adventures. I only ever thought of myself as an ordinary bloke. I still do.

Introduction

I've been a fighter since I was a young boy. Not actually fighting other people, at least not initially. What I mean is, when faced with difficulties and incredible odds stacked against me I didn't just give up. I dug deep and fought tooth and nail, and I came out on top of situations because I was always willing to go longer and harder than anyone else. I was driven by my desire to find security, structure and independence. At times this was to my detriment. I suffered a lot by completing so-called goals and objectives I thought were important at the time but feeling empty once I got there.

I had been struggling to make sense of life since I was a young boy. Some people can just accept their lot in life and never have the inner urge to seek a deeper understanding of life.

For me, I now feel deeply that I had no choice. As soon as I was old enough to know there were many unanswered questions about the nature of my existence, my journey began. It wasn't until I started to let go of trying to control the destiny of my journey and allowed life to guide me that I finally started to find peace.

When I was 17, and had had enough of the effects of being bullied, teased and down on myself throughout my childhood, I made a decision that would change my life and set me on a journey that would start to address some of my fears, insecurities and deeper questions like 'Who am I?' and 'What is my purpose?'. I left school, got a job and started martial arts. I truly believed martial arts was a vehicle for not only learning to fight but also the development of my spirit.

For as long as I can remember I have had a fascination with Japan. I remember when I was 11 years old, I was in primary school, and completed a school project on Japan. I was fascinated that such a small country was so powerful and had so many unique facets to its culture. My father had two full traditional pots of sake he brought back from Japan on one of his business trips. They intrigued me, and I was constantly looking at them and feeling the weight of the mysterious contents.

Pictures of the ancient samurai warrior set my imagination in motion, and took me on journeys to Japan in my dreams. They were dedicated to learning their art of war and protecting their master. Over time the samurai developed into a type of spiritual warrior, striving to perfect their martial arts skills and developing a deeper connection with nature. The samurai were a part of the ancient culture of Japan, and their influence on Japanese society continues to this day. I would eventually go on to live in Japan and immerse myself fully into Japanese life.

The following is a collection of individual experiences over a period of 35 years that may seem quite ordinary, but to me were very powerful and challenging in every way. These were not life or death experiences. Rather, they pushed me way out of my personal comfort zone without being negligent or careless. With the exception of a few spur-of-the-moment experiences, most were well thought out and carefully planned.

Even so, having said that, even with careful and meticulous planning, in the blink of an eye things could quickly get out of control and become very dangerous. The lesson for me is how I survived each experience and then related it to my personal growth.

Throughout my martial arts career there have always been injuries. Many training and sparring sessions were a fight for survival, so stopping because you took a few head shots or dislocated a toe was not an option. Small fractures to the fingers and toes, corked thighs and black eyes were the norm, and would be nursed with ice packs for a couple of hours at the most. Most injuries would heal themselves in a week or so, but it was common to be carrying chronic injuries for months. This was part of the way we developed spirit – we taped up the injury and kept training. We didn't run off to have an x-ray or see the physio unless it was very serious.

I used to think I got through the majority of my hard training years with minimum impact and injury to my body. But I know now that is not the case. Every significant bump or bruise is remembered by the body. Even though I now have chronic ankle and knee problems, I still manage to train every day and keep my body structure and old injuries managed by yoga, tai chi and chi gong.

I tried to avoid head contact to minimise the long-term damage to the brain. That is the main reason I did not enter competitions that allowed full head contact. But in the natural process of training I experienced a lot of head trauma. I have always had my strong physical exterior, power, flexibility and fighting nous, and the ability to dig deeper mentally and emotionally to be able to face up to and conquer whatever challenge had been placed in front of me.

It was the world that I existed in and relished. Though I was slowly transitioning to softer forms of training such as tai chi and chi gong (which are easier in the body) and regularly meditating, I still very much enjoyed sparring my top black belts every Saturday morning.

So when I began to slowly and insidiously lose my physical prowess, I reacted by training harder, sparring harder, and refusing to give in to the deeper fears that spurred on anxiety and depression that ate away at me. I knew something was not right, but lived in denial and found a sense of solace in the fact that medically no-one could find anything wrong with me.

As I began to struggle with washing my hair, tying my shoelaces and typing I adapted, and justified that I was okay because I could still do a strong sparring session with my senior black belts. But I was still in denial. My left punch, which had always been so sharp, tired quickly. So rather than just give in I trained myself to spar and fight on my other side. I refused to believe that my physical castle that I had taken so long to build into such a powerful force, and had for so long been the core of my being, was beginning to falter.

The neurologist was clinical in his testing, and I knew I was not performing well. I held my arms out, tapped my fingers, and made feeble attempts at other tests of dexterity. After about 10 minutes the specialist asked me to get dressed and take a seat. He looked at me, deep sorrow in his eyes.

'You have Parkinson's disease.'

This is not a story about my life with Parkinson's disease. As you will see, the Parkinson's disease is just part of a bigger picture of my life. It is about my initial struggle with life, and how my many teachers played an integral part in guiding me to recognise and eventually not be controlled by deep-seated fears, phobias and insecurities.

A diagnosis of Parkinson's disease, though potentially devastating, set me free and enabled me to finally live my life. This book is a message of hope, love and peace in that no matter what we are faced with in life and ultimately in death, living your truth – and I mean *really* living it – will guide you to a deeper understanding of who you are and, ultimately, peace.

Opposite page:
At my best at 27 years of age.

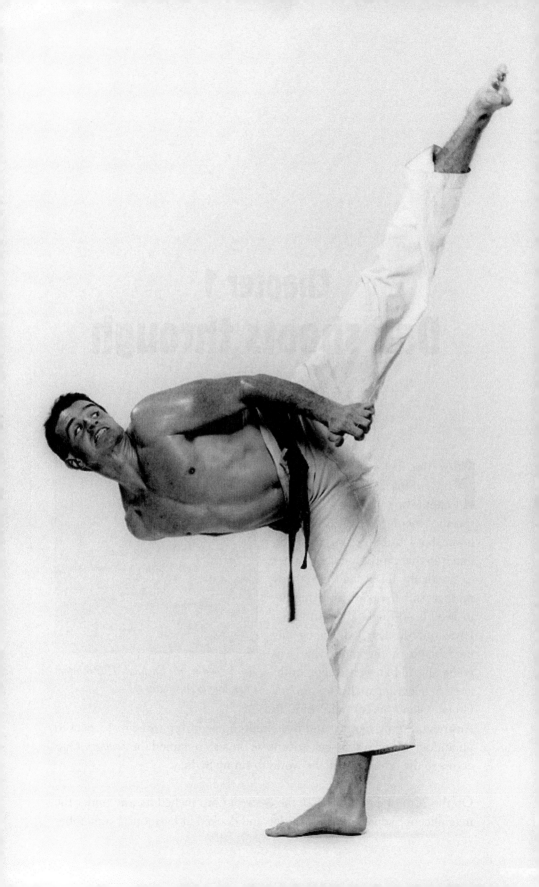

Chapter 1

Protection through

Chapter 1
Dad shoots through

For the first five years of my life I think I was a normal and happy boy. I do not have any specific memories of friction at home, but I am sure it was there. So much so that it prompted my father to suddenly up it and leave my mother and five kids and migrate in 1969 from England to Australia. I was only five, so I did not really understand at the time what was going on. All I knew was six months later a telegram arrived from my father asking us to join him in Australia. So my mother and five children aged from three to 13 packed up and set sail on a six-week adventure on a ship named the *Southern Cross* across to the other side of the world to sunny Sydney.

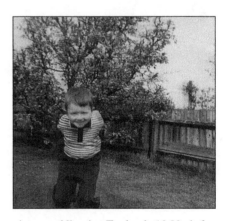

As a toddler in England 1969 before migrating to Australia.

On the 26th of January 1970, the *Southern Cross* inched its way under the magnificent Sydney Harbour bridge and docked in Pyrmont. I remember seeing my father waving as the large ship moored and dropped anchor. I was excited at the thought of seeing Dad, but I did not really know him. The sky was clear and blue, the kind of day that Sydney is famous for. Dad loaded us all into his new white Holden stationwagon and we headed off to one of Sydney's furthest suburbs, Berowra. The old house backed onto the edge of the bush, which turned out to be great, especially for three young boys. We got to know and enjoy the bush, and even now I have a great love of Australian nature.

After dropping me and my brothers and sisters at the house in Berowra, Dad and my mother went for a drive. On that drive, my father asked my mother for a divorce. What followed were years and years of anger, sorrow and pain that my mother, my brothers and sisters and I all had to work through in our own way and find peace with. There is no doubt that what happened between my mother and father has had a profound effect on all our lives.

Band of brothers

I often think of my mother who passed away a couple of years ago, and wonder where she is. We were close in many ways, but the fear was always there. Not in a physical way, but rather emotionally. She would turn in an instant from being incredibly kind to angry and nasty. I never really had any idea how it was going to be at home.

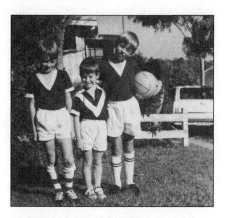

Early life in Berowra in Sydney. L-R: me, my younger brother John, and my older brother Robin.

My sisters were older and claimed their independence from a young age. I don't have any clear memories of living with my sisters. My brothers and I lived our lives constantly walking on eggshells, but we had each other. The three of us were a band of brothers, and we found solace in the great adventures we had exploring the Australian bush directly behind our home in the outer suburb of Berowra and making it our own. It was in many ways an escape from the continued on-again, off-again drama going on between Mum and Dad.

As brothers, we played war games, continually dodging the bull ant nests and having fun experimenting with homemade bombs made from the gunpowder of firecrackers that were legal when we were kids. It's a wonder we never lost a finger or an eye.

I was fascinated by the strangeness and uniqueness of the Australian bush. Things like the laughing kookaburra, the tawny frogmouth birds, and the frilled neck lizards that would let you get so close that one of us would lob a rock at it to see if it was still alive, laughing as it would make a bolt for the bush on its two hind legs. We knew where the best ponds were, and we would catch fat yabbies and cook them in a billy of boiling water. I even learned to sleep and be comforted by the monotonous shrill of the summer cicada.

White skin and freckles

We arrived at Berowra Public School to what we thought was the first day of term. But Mum, trying to juggle the first day of school for five kids, got it very wrong. We were a day late. Mum dropped me at the school gate and I had to find my own way to the school's office. I was six years old and having to fend for myself in a new school, new city and new country.

At first, they did not know what to do with me. They weren't expecting me, so I sat in between two classrooms for the day while they sorted it out. I was so self-conscious

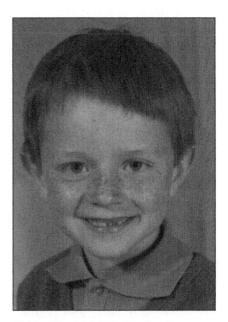

White-skinned and freckle-faced.

as all the children from both classrooms pointed and giggled.

I was a shy boy with white skin, freckles and a large cowlick that flicked up my fringe. I had an English accent that caught the attention of not only the girls but also the older boys who were keen on the girls. So from very early on I was a target.

Now I know that many of us were bullied and/or teased in school. And I'm not saying it was any worse for me. But the whole situation was compounded by my home situation. After the divorce, Mum was desperately unhappy and cried a lot. She really wanted to return to England, but had no money or place to call home. The entire situation was made worse as Dad, though divorced, continued to skirt around the edges – coming and going, playing happy families one minute, leaving the next. Not giving Mum space to heal, and not really giving his sons the attention they so desperately yearned for.

Being bullied with the constant threat of violence left me alone and confused. Back then as a six-year-old I did not know what bullying was. I just knew I wasn't liked by the older boys, so any self-esteem and confidence were quickly eroded.

There was one older boy. His name was John Duggan. He would taunt me to fight him in front of the girls. I remember it was a Friday afternoon, and I was heading to the school gate to go home when I was confronted by Duggan. In front of a group of girls, Duggan challenged me to a fight. Naturally I said 'No' and started to cry as I had no idea what to do. One of the older girls stepped in to protect me, but Duggan kept on calling me a 'limey chicken'.

From somewhere deep inside I spoke. I agreed to fight him on the Monday morning in the school playground. I learned from a young age the power of words and managed to manipulate a compromise. That entire weekend I was in various states of fear, and felt very alone.

Monday morning came, and I felt like a condemned man waiting for the end. But I put one foot in front of the other and made my way towards the school yard. It was empty. I waited. Duggan did not turn up, and I never saw him again.

These incidents from a young age slowly set a blueprint of fear and uncertainty in me that were reinforced by my parents' inability to parent their children. I was a very scared, self-conscious boy who lacked any trace of confidence or self-esteem. The perfect target for bullies.

Home was not a happy place. My therapist says that when my parents divorced in 1970, which was a long drawn-out affair, I lost the ability to feel. I mean I can conceptualise feeling, but not actually feel. I removed that capacity out of the need to protect myself from the emotional rollercoaster ride I went through because of my mother's unpredictable moods.

Not feeling does not mean that I did not care. The problem was that I cared too much. I was a very sensitive child, and I worried about everything from a very young age. Trying to explain how I felt about the situation at home was always very difficult. I just behaved in a manner that would make Mum happy despite how I really felt inside. So by the time I was ready to set off into the world, I was quite shut off emotionally.

High school dropout

I was not a born fighter. In fact, I was the complete opposite. Other than wrestling with my brothers I did not have a clue how to defend myself. When reading this you may wonder why I didn't just lash out, but I didn't know that was an option. No-one told me. My childhood did everything it possibly could to remove any chance of having a positive male role model in my life who could guide me as a good father guides a son.

I had a mother who tried her best, but was and remained bitter her entire life by the departure of my father. And though she tried hard, she never failed at shaming me in front of my friends throughout my childhood. My friends were constantly being reprimanded by my mother for not addressing her correctly, and I would sink to the floor with embarrassment every time it happened.

In 1973, when we moved from Berowra to Normanhurst, my mother dressed me in the Normanhurst High School uniform and not the primary school uniform I was supposed to wear. At lunchtime the other children teased and taunted me, calling me a high school dropout. Not a great first day at my new school.

It was these kinds of incidents that compounded and reinforced my very low opinion of myself.

After that initial embarrassment, I settled in and made new friends and things were going well. At the beginning of Year 5 a new teacher by the name of Mr Panic, a larger-than-life man with a brash and aggressive personality, arrived to teach. He was the exact opposite of what I needed at that stage of my life, and he soon singled me out as an easy target.

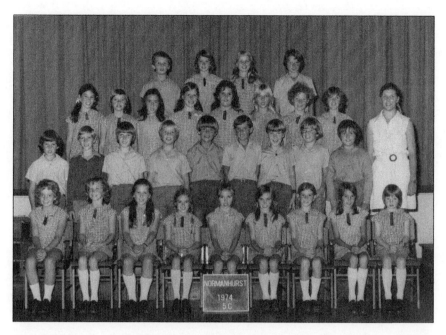

I am in the top row, far right-hand side. Mrs Crampton, my Year 5 teacher, is on the right.

He did not teach me directly, as there were two Year 5 classes. But he got to know me through the drama classes and sport, both of which I was starting to excel at. In many ways he was similar to my mother only way scarier, especially for an 11-year-old who would attach to any feedback from an alpha male.

He was kind and full of praise one minute, but would turn and completely strip me of any confidence the moment I made a mistake or slipped up. Mr Panic was the rugby coach, and because I was becoming a fast runner I had some success playing rugby. I dropped the ball from a high kick once, and Mr Panic labelled me 'butter fingers'. He would take every opportunity to tease and humiliate me in front of the other boys. To this day, I still do not have the confidence to catch a rugby ball from a high kick.

In Year 5 I was selected to be the lead part of 'The Flying Pieman' in the play by the same name. I was so proud, and the play was a great success. For once I enjoyed the attention. It felt good. When the time came to choose the parts for the next play, I was not considered and left out completely. When I asked Mr Panic why, he yelled and screamed at me, taunting me to tell him why I should be included. He reduced me to tears.

At morning tea time Mr Panic was on playground duty, and so I remained in my classroom as I was too afraid to see him. Mrs Crampton, my teacher, was also very upset by seeing how distraught I was. She said that she would speak to him and sort things out.

In the end I was given a bit part in the play band. He dressed me up in a traditional German Oktoberfest leather jumpsuit, and put me right at the front of the stage. Everyone but me thought it was a great laugh. I was totally alone. I remember these experiences vividly because they had such a lasting impact on me.

I just kept on going. I kept on showing up and trying my hardest to fit in and be accepted. Back then I had no idea of resilience or spirit, but deep down I felt that just giving up was not an option. It never has been, and it never will be. Over the years I have attempted to explain this quality of not giving up when things get tough but have found it hard.

I think everyone has a breaking point, and that some can endure more than others. It is what you do and how you feel once you *do* give up that is important. Not giving up as soon as the going gets tough is a champion quality that creates resilience and self-discipline. And the more you do it, the better you get at it.

Even now, as I wake each morning I am quickly reminded by the pulsating shaking of my hand of the challenge I now face each day. I am not defined by Parkinson's disease. It simply adds a new dimension to my life, and I am adjusting to accommodate it.

I went on in Year 6 to become vice-captain and school athletics and swimming champion at Normanhurst Primary School. I also passed the entry test into James Ruse, one of Australia's top academic high schools.

Fear will always be there. It will justify itself in so many ways. Sometimes it is good. It will protect you. Other times it will stop you from living a vital and fulfilling life. See it, feel it, observe it, then work back and try to see the cause. When you have that, then work back again and again. It's interesting when we finally understand what the real reason for the fear is.

The Apple Tree Bay incident

The one incident that stands out above all others was when I was 13 and finishing my first year at James Ruse High School. A handful of my schoolmates and I set off on a hike from Mt Kuring-gai Station to Apple Tree Bay, a beautiful and popular swimming spot on the Hawkesbury River just north of Sydney.

The day was warm, and we were all looking forward to jumping off the high rock into the cool water. We had been swimming for about an hour when another group of older boys we did not know arrived and took the benches close to us. It wasn't long before they started to throw taunts at us. We were a small bunch of selective school nerds, and it soon became obvious to our new tormentors that we were an easy target as we did not initially respond to their abuse.

I remember them walking past us to the steps to the river and we all looked away as they scowled at us. They were busting for a fight, and one boy in particular stood out from the others. I was scared and ashamed that I looked away as his rant continued. At last they were past us and swimming. But the taunts continued. Because I thought the threat was over I found my voice and responded with a witty comment that made us all laugh. But the aggressive one did not find it funny at all. He flipped out and swam directly to the steps, and before I knew it was standing in front of me demanding an apology. Next thing I knew was smash – he king hit me on the side of the face.

'Fight me,' he screamed.

Smash, smash and again smash as he pummelled my face with left and right punches. I just remained sitting on the bench stunned, taking his punches, unable to move. None of us could.

This fine young gentleman exhausted himself by using me as a punching bag. I wasn't physically hurt, though my jaw ached for a couple of days. But I was at a complete loss as to why I did not defend myself. I think back now and realise that it was such a random and bizarre event, and I was in no way prepared for it.

But it did not finish there. After he finished with me, he and his mates returned to their bench. We packed our bags and made our way past their group. They took great delight in calling me a chicken (slang for coward) as I passed by, and I was utterly ashamed of myself.

We made our way up the hill and along the narrow bush track, and from below their abuse continued. We could all hear 'Your mate is a chicken shit' being yelled up at us. Silly me yelled back, hoping to at least gain a morsel of any respect left from my mates.

Before I knew it, he had run up the hill and caught up to us. The assault continued, with him punching me in the face. I slipped on the loose ground, landing on my back. He was over me in an instant. But then something inside me switched on and I lashed out, kicking upward and catching him right on the chest.

It shocked him, and that one strike out by me stunned and hurt him. I had taken 20 or more of his punches and was not hurt. One kick from me and he gave up. He stopped and stood back, a look of hesitation and fear. I almost laughed at the sight of his skin marked by a big red imprint of my foot. He went quiet and retreated down the hill. And that was that.

Iron jaw

The ordeal at Apple Tree Bay haunted me for many years. Over time I came to realise it was not being hit that traumatised me. Although one good thing came out of the ordeal: I knew I had an iron jaw. It was the sheer humiliation of being hit so many times myself in front of mates and not defending myself, and later thinking I was a coward. Some may see that I actually won in the end, but I have never seen it that way.

It was a driving force that would propel me into as many situations as possible to prove to myself that I was not a coward. I struggled through high school, keeping my head down and avoiding any confrontation. The Apple Tree Bay incident was not talked about at school by my friends or to my family. But the scars were always there, just below the surface. At Apple Tree Bay my innocence and childlike wonder of the world had been brutally ripped from under me, and I was left fibrillating awkwardly as I tried desperately to regain a foothold of reality. In the remaining years at school I suffered chronic insomnia as a result of the constant emotional blackmail and tension that my mother put on me as I attempted to pursue a relationship with my father. I also felt a relentless pressure from the school to excel academically, and this only added to my distress.

Touched by an angel

For as long as I can remember I have been aware of a gap left by a childhood with no significant male role models to guide me. As a child I both yearned for and feared strong men, loving the attention when I got it but being repelled by their anger or passive aggression.

I was 13 years old before any man paid me any attention that was worth anything. Keith Knight, who lived across the road from us in Normanhurst with his family, was the local scout master. My older brother and I had been members of scouts for a couple of months when one evening Keith took me aside and sat me down. And what he said changed my life.

He said, 'Young man, I see you walking up and down the path, looking down towards the ground, your shoulders all hunched over, afraid to look at anyone. Lift your head up, stand tall, put your shoulders back and look up into this beautiful world. You have the incredible potential to achieve anything you want in life.'

I lapped up everything he said. I changed the way I walked, and it changed the way I looked at the world. Those few words touched me, and I have never forgotten them.

Chapter 2
Philosophy training

I n 1980, when I started to become interested in martial arts, I did not know very much about what it consisted of other than watching Bruce Lee in his now famous movies in the early 1970s. Initially seeing his movies as a young boy, I was moved that Bruce used his skills as the protector and doer of what was just and good.

After enjoying the Bruce Lee movies, I was then mesmerised by the all-knowing Master Po, the blind warrior monk in the 1970s television series *Kung Fu* starring the late actor David Carradine as his disciple. Master Po espoused a beautiful philosophy, strict ethics and a code of conduct to his disciple Kane during his time at the Shaolin Temple.

From the age of 10, my early exposure to the martial arts was quite powerful in that I was able to absorb even at a young age that there was more to martial arts than just kicking and punching. There was a deeper philosophy. So when I first took an interest in learning martial arts at 17, it was understandable that I had visions of quickly finding a master who could catapult me physically and spiritually to a greater understanding of myself. Little did I know that ideal and belief would take me on an incredible journey.

At its core, many people train in martial arts because it represents training for a greater purpose, not just to learn how to fight. Ordinary people are not necessarily interested in sparring or competing in tournaments. They are more interested in the confidence, self-esteem and feeling of wellbeing that can be gained from learning the physical techniques of any martial art. I soon understood these great benefits but wanted more.

So it was in the martial arts that my journey began. But I was looking for the perfection in a master, which I came to realise was impossible. No matter what level you are at, there are always parts of us that need to be worked on. True mastery begins by being aware what those flaws are and then learning ways to renew ourselves every day, and not just existing on autopilot.

Mr Clatworthy makes a prediction

Year 10 at high school could not come fast enough. I was 16, and I'd decided immediately that I would finish my schooling early and attempt to leave all the demons behind as soon as I could. I wanted my independence as soon as possible. I thought that training as a tradesman, although physically challenging, would enable me to quickly establish my own business, giving me for the first time an element of control over my life.

At the same time as commencing my apprenticeship, I was walking around to my car at the old side of Hornsby station when a poster in a hairdresser's window caught my eye. There was this Asian man flying through the air delivering the most amazing kick. I was captivated. It was a poster for the local taekwondo school. So one evening I headed to the Waitara community centre for what would be a life-changing experience.

The instant I walked into the class I knew I was home. I cannot begin to explain the feeling. It was not that I was excited. It was that I was totally at ease, and the martial arts had been waiting for me to make the discovery. I realised in that instant that if I had not suffered the way I did at school, I never would have had the inclination to look at something like taekwondo.

I loved it, and it loved me. We fitted each other like a glove. I devoted myself to training, quickly learning the skills and learning how to fight. At the same time, I was starting to see new muscle and strength from all the manual labour at work. It was not long until I was starting to fight and beat the senior students in my taekwondo class.

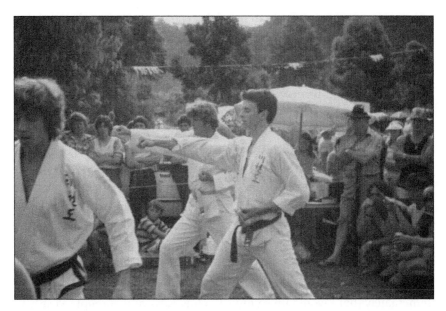

A blue belt in taekwondo at a demonstration at Wisemans Ferry in 1981. I was 18 years old. My first instructor, Master Tim Hassall, is front left.

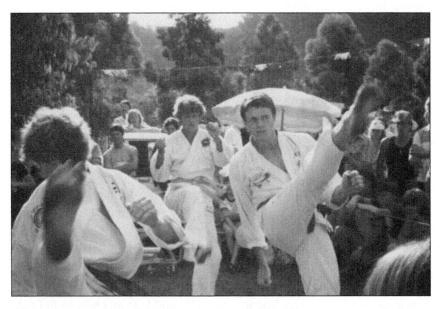

Kicking as a Blue Belt. There was a certain intensity in my technique from early on.

Emerging from Year 10 at 16 years old, I was thrust into the male domain of the blue-collar workforce. Back in 1979, when I left school, it was generally thought that you left in Year 10 because you were not academic and entering into an apprenticeship was your only option. At the end of Year 10 at James Ruse, not only did I receive a distinction in mathematics, but also a high distinction in art and credits in all other subjects.

So despite my difficulties with stress and anxiety during high school, I finished with remarkable results. So much so that the maths master Mr Clatworthy remarked with astonishment in front of the class that he guaranteed I would be back to finish my schooling within 12 months.

Though he was wrong, and I did not go back to school, I was soon to learn that my level of education was unique among the men I encountered during my early years as an apprentice plumber and the other boys I met at trade school. I recognised this very early in my apprenticeship, and although it created doubt in my mind as to whether this path was right for me, I pushed any thought of quitting out of my mind and blindly pushed on and through the torment inflicted on me by my uneducated fellow workers. Though I knew deep down this choice of career did not suit me, because of my ability to be able to endure all kinds of hardship I was determined to survive all that I was subjected to and complete the six years required to become a licensed plumber.

Practice determination – the ability to go beyond your perceived barriers. The belief that you can succeed regardless of your current situation. Use the small wins in life to prepare you for the big challenges. Sometimes, from the depths of despair a tiny flicker of hope is enough to help you put one foot in front of the other. Challenge yourself constantly by facing your fears.

The boy

Being a first-year apprentice on a construction site, I was the bottom of the pecking order. I was referred to as 'the boy'. It was always, 'Boy, go and get me this,' or 'Boy, go and get me that'. Not only was I responsible for collecting the morning tea and lunch orders, I was also the general topic of all jokes and pranks. The other tradesmen would think nothing would be funnier than holding me down and spray painting my legs green.

At Canterbury racecourse, where I worked building a new grandstand, there was a large and deep grease trap. (Grease traps are used to catch the grease and sludge that is washed down sinks in restaurants.) The one at the racecourse collected the grease from the restaurants, and every couple of weeks it had to be cleaned. This involved climbing down a ladder into the trap and shovelling the grease into a bucket.

The first and last time I cleaned it, I passed the bucket full of thick putrid grease up to Peter Smith, a plumber, only to have the entire contents of the bucket tipped back onto my head. It was in my hair and dripping off my nose. I cleaned myself up as best I could, but still had to wear the same clothes stinking of foul cooking grease for the remainder of the day.

Plumbers have to deal with some of the worst working conditions, and being the apprentice meant I had to do some pretty filthy jobs. Jim Reynolds, the supervisor of the plumbing team at the racecourse, and I were assigned a week's work renewing a collapsed drainage pipe at a block of units in Sydney's leafy northern suburb of Killara. I was looking forward to the break from the other plumbers and I liked Jim.

As soon as we arrived at the block of units I quickly summed up the reason I was assigned to this job. There was a large hole in the front garden full of excrement, toilet paper and mud. The drainage pipe that connects the main sewerage network to the property is called the shaft. Sometimes, when there has been a leak because a pipe leading to the shaft is old, the ground around the pipe collapses, causing the pipe to break apart. Naturally, the people living in the unit block keep using their bathrooms and kitchens. But instead of the waste going down the sewerage pipe, it just collects in a huge seething pit of human waste until the plumbers arrive.

Jim had a wry smile on his face as he threw me a bucket and shovel and said, 'It's all yours, boy' as he made himself comfortable with a smoke and the newspaper well way from the stench.

The hardest thing about cleaning out the pit was no matter how many times we asked the residents not to use the toilet, excrement kept flowing down into the pit. Jim could see my frustration, and said he knew a trick that would help. He would go and tell the residents again not to use their toilets. In the meantime he told me to put my ear up to the pipe leading to the pit from the units (the pipe end was at head height in the pit), and when I heard the water coming to put a bucket up to the pipe and catch it before it filled the pit again. I totally trusted Jim, so there was no reason to think this was another prank.

I never heard the water coming down the pipe. There was an eerie silence, but I waited and diligently listened. I wanted to show Jim that he could trust me to get the job done.

I heard the rush, but it was all too late. The excrement filled my ear, my hair and I was literally in the shit from head to toe. As Jim arrived back he could not hold back his laughter as he threw me a towel. It was then that I realised it was him who had used the toilet.

Apart from Keith Knight from my scouts group, and a couple of other sporadic acts of male kindness up until I was in my early twenties, I'd never experienced other men behaving in any other way other than to bully or humiliate me. With Dad not around that much while I was growing up, this was what I knew.

> *The hardest skill to learn in martial arts is killer instinct. This skill needs to be nurtured by the teacher a little at a time. Killer instinct is not angry or aggressive. It is cold and unemotional. The martial artist who has honed their killer instinct is still and neutral in combat.*

Bullied for the last time

I was working on the new grandstand at Canterbury racecourse, and company bully Peter Smith would single me out at every opportunity to make himself look funny at my expense. I quietly put up with it, but I was no longer the scared schoolboy. I was growing into a man. Training daily at taekwondo and pushing myself hard at work, I had metamorphosed into a 183cm, 90kg ball of muscle and sinew.

And I could fight.

As my strength built, Smith didn't notice. It crept up on him, and I took my time and waited for the perfect opportunity. I did not have to wait long. Our lunch room was in a large white caravan set up as an office and tea room for the team of plumbers. We finished lunch, and stood up to go back to work. Smith pushed me in the back and said, 'Hurry up, boy' as I left the caravan. I fell down the stairs, ending up head first in a pile of rubbish. Everyone laughed. Smith thought it was hilarious, but he did not see the look on my face. It was one of those times in life when you just know you have had enough and life will never be the same again.

From a crouching position I leapt up and was onto Smith in the blink of an eye. I had him by the shirt with both hands and drove him up and back so hard that his back hit the wall with a thud. I lifted him by the shirt so that he was off the ground. I then looked him squarely in the eyes and said to him that if he ever put a hand on me again I would beat the shit out of him.

He was petrified. I never had any trouble from him again. In fact, that was the last time anyone has laid a hand on me without my permission. This was the first time in my life that I found the courage to stand up for myself. It was the day I went from being a boy to a man. I had found and recognised a part of me that had always been there but never nurtured, and I did it without any help.

A taste of spirituality

At around the time I commenced taekwondo, I picked up an old thin hardback book on meditation out of my mother's bookcase. I looked through it, and although I did not understand a word of what it was saying, I had the feeling that meditation for me was something I needed to learn more about. I started to devour a whole range of self-help books starting with *Creative Visualisation* by Shakti Gawain and *Jonathan Livingston Seagull* by Richard Bach. As I finished one, another would jump off the bookshelf – books by Leo Buscaglia, Wayne Dyer, Shirley MacLaine and Elizabeth Kubler Ross to name a few. Then there was the famous book *Way of the Peaceful Warrior* by Dan Millman, which I enjoyed immensely.

At the time, I did not know quite what I was looking for. But the books made me feel good, and whet my appetite for more. Looking back now, I can see that this was the beginning of my spiritual path. I was also keen to learn how to meditate, so when I was 20 I found a great meditation group called Friends of the Western Buddhist Society in George St, Sydney. Unfortunately, though I loved the meditation at the time, I did not keep it up. I was not ready, and it would be many years before it would make a significant impact on my life.

Never underestimate the power of personal intention. When who we are aligns with what we are, mountains can be moved. When you can feel yourself in a flow, and there is no struggle or resistance, you are following your true path and purpose.

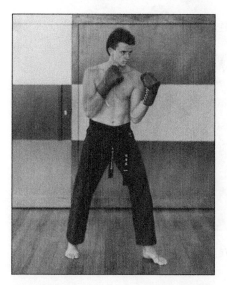

Me, just after I was awarded a black belt.

The teacher

From the time I was awarded my first black belt at 21 I commenced teaching. My first school was at Hiscoes Gym and Squash Centre in Surry Hills. I did not have any plans as to how martial arts would go on to play such a large part in my life. It just felt good to do something I was good at, so I continued to do it. I taught taekwondo to both kids and adults, and trained for competitions. Back then the new sport of kickboxing was all the rage, and other than taekwondo and karate competitions there was not much around competition-wise. I met long-time mates Dimi Tops and Mark Russell through early karate competitions. We would meet and train in Goju karate, kickboxing and taekwondo. They were rough and dangerous sessions, with regular knockouts and other injuries. The so-called 'no-contact sparring' took on new meaning. After being punched in the face several times, I soon came to understand that in those days 'no-contact' meant fast and furious fighting with little or no regard for rules.

At 22, as well as teaching at Hiscoes during the week, I was keen to test my skills against other local styles of martial arts. So I commenced an open sparring class in the HCF Gym in Chatswood on Saturday afternoons. The class attracted many different styles of martial arts, and as I expected was put to the test many times.

There were top fighters such as Mike Kenworthy (full-contact karate) and Colin Handley (heavyweight taekwondo champion), as well as numerous kung fu, hapkido and Wing Chun devotees, boxers, and people who just loved to test themselves. Many times I had to fight for my survival. But

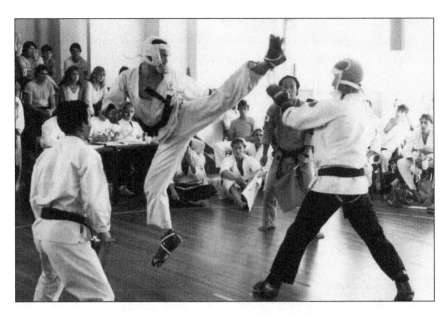

At an early karate tournament in Bondi. It was here that many long-term friendships were made.

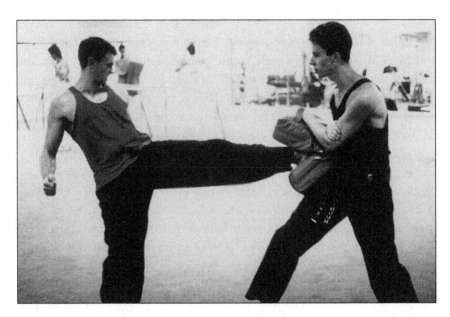

Kicking the bag, held by my brother John at HCF Gym at Chatswood.

it was during these times that I did my combat apprenticeship. I bashed many fighters, but also got my fair share of bashings in return. Every Saturday night I had to ice injuries and nurse bruises, and I would limp for days after.

Attaining a black belt, you have shown great commitment and dedication to achieving an end result, a set goal. How you then go on and apply being a black belt in everyday life will determine the kind of black belt you will become.

One Saturday, when I was 23, I had to take the afternoon off from HCF as I was competing in a taekwondo competition. I ended up winning after a couple of tough bouts, and spent the night in hospital with a dislocated knuckle. My girlfriend at the time liked to attend the Saturday afternoon sessions, and my younger brother John was always there to supervise.

On this particular Saturday afternoon the class was visited by a rather angry bodybuilder who was also a very good fighter. I had known him for years, and watched him go from a very classy martial artist into a nasty thug massively juiced up on steroids. I avoided him, but I knew we were on a collision course to meet sooner or later. It just so happened that he came looking for me the day I was competing.

He went on to hurt most of the students that day, including dislocating my girlfriend Mary's shoulder. I did not find any of this out until I checked out of hospital the following morning. I was keen to get some payback, but with my hand out of action I was in no shape to do any kind of fighting.

I waited until the swelling in my hand had gone down enough so I could put a boxing glove on. I then contacted the bodybuilder, and he agreed to meet me in the main hall at Harbord Diggers Club, just north of Manly Beach. This was not intended to be a malicious grudge match. There was no anger, just two fighters challenging their ability.

He moved quickly and smoothly, immediately landing a straight hard left punch that shook me and dropped me to one knee. I got up quickly, a little shaken and surprised. I recovered quickly, launching a wave of kicks aimed at his head. He easily slipped my kicks and stunned me with a powerful low kick to my left leg that hurt me and slowed me down. I backed off to regroup, then feinted a straight left jab to his head and followed immediately with a left side kick aimed at his stomach. He winced as the side kick found its mark. I did not hesitate and quickly countered, launching him across the room with my signature spinning back kick, cracking several of his ribs. He was doubled over in pain, but he was still able put his hand out to indicate he did not want to continue.

The entire episode was no longer than a minute. One of us was going down that morning, and I was determined it was not going to be me.

There are plenty of people who are nothing more than scared boys hiding behind an angry aggressive front. Get these bullies one on one and put a little pressure on, and you soon see their true colours.

Chapter 3
The nightclub door

No matter how much I trained in martial arts, and no matter how many different competitions I entered, I still felt the shame and effects of bullying like a shadow hanging over me. I decided that a great way to prove to myself that I was okay and not a coward was to expose myself to potential situations where I would be forced to either talk my way out of it or defend myself. Without going out and picking fights on the street, I thought working the nightclub door was a sensible option.

When someone pushes, move aside and let them pass. This takes strength of mind as your previous action would be to resist, make a point, or have a compulsive need to give your opinion. This attitude saved me many times on the door.

The Scottish rugby team

The first night I worked as a bouncer was in the early eighties. At that time, Jameson St nightclub was probably the place to be seen when discos were at their peak. I did not need the money as I was working full time. I was just really keen to put myself under pressure to see how I would react. I was 22 years old, a black belt, and could handle myself pretty well, or so I thought. I was sure that if it came down to it my fighting skills would get me out of trouble and I was so ready. Naïve, but ready.

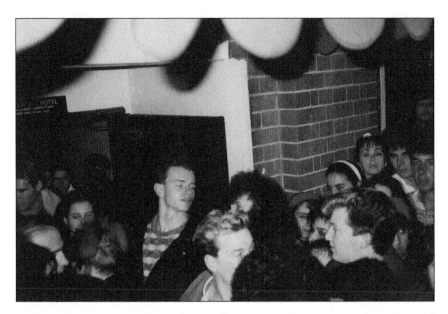

Berlin Club. Jameson St Nightclub on a Tuesday night. I am in front of the door with my head turned. Robert and Paul are on the far left.

My first night started, and the flow of people in and out of the club was smooth. It was a busy Tuesday night at the popular Berlin Club, and I was a little green to say the least. Customers come up to the door, you check them out, and if they look okay you unclip the rope and let them in.

Hey, this is easy, I thought. *No trouble here.*

There were three of us on the door that night: Paul, an experienced bouncer and kind of a De Niro lookalike who was small but looked like he could hold his own, Robert, who is now a well-known actor, and me. Paul and Robert were in the club having a walk through and I was on the door alone for the first time.

In an instant, my confident air of invincibility was shattered. I was confronted by several huge Scottish footballers (wearing kilts and all) who were in Australia to take on the Wallabies rugby team. Four of them towered over me as I stood behind the flimsy rope barrier. I felt alone and very, very vulnerable. They were drunk, charged up and looking for a fight. I was an easy target for them. And on top of that, trying to understand a drunken Scotsman can be difficult at the best of times.

I said 'No' to their constant demands to enter the club. This just enraged them even more. Paul and Robert were quickly back at my side, checking what all the commotion was about. Paul, the shorter one of us, quickly became aggressive and started shouting. The last I saw of Paul that night was him being set upon and tossed around like a rugby ball amongst the Scots. I turned and looked for support from Robert, and the last I saw of him was his back as he closed the front door behind him, leaving me to handle the Scots myself.

Talk about being thrown into the deep end.

Six of them moved towards me. They picked up the rope barrier and supports, and hurled them up the street. The large crowd that was waiting to get into the club was silent.

Okay, Andy. You asked for it. Now let's see what you have got.

I had no place to run. They had me trapped between the inside door and the front door. I resigned myself to having to fight it out.

I readied myself and became still, unemotional as I steadied the terror that was churning within me. The first footballer came towards me, and just for an instant I could feel the hesitation in him. He came steaming into me with a round kick to my leg. I could see it coming a mile away, so I just slid back out of the way. As he came through he lost balance and slipped. I moved, and he landed in a big heap in front of me. I remained still and silent. Nothing needed to be done or said. Two of the other Scots quickly came in, picked up their mate, looked at me, and to my surprise said, 'Sorry mate' as they turned and quickly made their way up the street.

> *Whatever you put out there will come back to you. If you are aggressive, you will get that in return. Your absolute best defence is 'still observation'.*

In the face of this assault, I did not need to do anything. My still, neutral presence said it all. I was ready to go all the way. Yes I was scared, but there was a deeper presence that came through me that was immediately felt by the attacker.

From the moment I commenced working at nightclubs, I knew I was in for an interesting experience. By nature I am not an aggressive person, and I don't look for trouble. But sometimes when you're working a door trouble just comes to you.

The only reason I worked on the door or as a bouncer was to gain people experience, and to put myself in dangerous situations that would challenge me mentally, physically and emotionally. I just needed to see how I would handle myself under pressure, see how I would react, and see if my training would survive in the street. I have many fond memories of that time in my life, but it also really opened my eyes to one of the ugly sides of partying.

Now, I am not the kind of person who goes around picking fights, or even reacts with aggression when I am picked on. So the next best option I thought was to get experience as a bouncer.

I must say from the start that even though the shift started at 8pm and finished at 4am, looking back I loved my entire time there. The team I worked with were mainly actors, musicians and models, and in between the crowds, the drunks and the police, did it test me? Well, yes. I was put into numerous situations where I had to remain calm and centred. I quickly learned this was always the best option.

With a little savvy and experience, I started to learn who to let into the clubs and who not to. I generally tended to avoid suits from the stock exchange across the road and others who looked of the legal variety. I don't know how many times I was threatened with, 'I will sue you, your family and your dog if you don't let me into the club'.

Suits

One Thursday night I was asked if I could work a private function at the club. I agreed because they usually paid well and were usually quiet. This night I was the only bouncer at a function for 100 stock traders—lovely gentlemen who just hated, and I mean *hated*, being told what to do. When I arrived at work the party was just getting started. It was my worst fear: the entire main bar was full of drunk stock traders. And it was not long before I was being harassed for kindly requesting them to take it easier on the drinks.

By the time the party was over the hardest part of the night is getting everyone to leave in a civil manner. 'Sir, the club closed an hour ago. It's time to leave.' As one group of about ten stock traders was leaving the club, they turned on me and got very aggressive. They were quite drunk and took a dislike to the way I was looking at them. But seriously, the entire night was just waiting to explode. By that stage of the night most were just pushing and shoving and all talk. In fact, what I found was the louder the voice the smaller the ticker. And very few men really knew how to handle themselves let alone throw a decent punch.

As the most violent of the group started to make a move on me, I raised my hands and cocked my leg to throw a side kick. It was clear that talking was over. I was fully prepared to fight, and to hurt as many of them as possible. Every ounce of my being was ready to hammer a side kick into the first man who came into range.

This is it, the essence of combat. When you are fully prepared to go all the way, it just oozes out of you. You set your target with a laser-like focus and it hits your attacker and stops him in his tracks. The attitude of the stock traders changed immediately. All of a sudden I was not such an easy target. They went very quiet and made their way from the club. Naturally I was relieved. This was an attitude I would take with me into many more confronting situations.

The moment you react you are drawing your sword. If you draw the sword, you had better be prepared to go all the way. Stop, breathe, become present, and respond with the knowledge of what is happening now, not what you have experienced in the past.

Girls' night

Friday night was girls' night, and some of my busiest nights were working the Hens parties on a Friday night. The ladies were entertained by male strippers and shirtless barmen. The shift started at 7pm, and it got busy from the beginning. The ladies were usually quite drunk early in the night. Strippers and alcohol do not make a good mix. We generally had to protect the strippers from being mobbed. Ladies would enjoy the male strippers until 11pm, then we would open the doors for the men to come in.

Anger has no prejudice. Quite often it would turn violent as we had to remove 'out of control' ladies. I have been assaulted by more women than I can care to remember. I was regularly covered in someone's drink. And I am proud to say I was always careful and diplomatic and remained cool.

One night a drunk woman threw a glass of champagne over me and grabbed my shirt. She was strong, and I knew she had a good grip. Striking her to release the grip would have quickly escalated the situation. I had to think fast. I ended up taking my shirt off. The last I saw of the woman and my shirt was her stumbling away from the club.

All in a night's work.

Keep your hands up

Sometimes the biggest danger in working as a bouncer/doorman comes not from the clientele but the other bouncers. This was back in the day when there was no regulation of the security industry, and you did not need a security license to work a door. So you never really knew the background of the person working beside you. You just hoped they would have your back.

Funny thing was, most of the other bouncers I worked with were all talk as well. I will never forget Gavin's first night on the door. Nice guy, good talker and remained cool. All that was great, but you also needed someone who was going to watch your back if the heat was on. I was not sure about Gav, a high-level Ninjutsu student. Now please, I have nothing against our Ninja brothers and sisters. But I did not want him to disappear in a puff of smoke if the brawl was on.

Gav did not last long. He took a swinging right hand and forgot the most basic of basic self-defence moves: keep your hands up.

Sometimes it was the other bouncers I had to protect myself against, or rather protect myself against their stupidity. At the front of the club there was a short hallway that can be closed at the street and another door from inside, effectively sealing the hallway. When there was a brawl at the door the internal door would be closed, quickly barricading the door against the brawl spilling into the club. We would then call the police and let them sort it out.

One night there was a fight on the door. Just a couple of drunks getting upset because I would not let them into the club. The other doormen were patrolling the club, so I was alone on the door. The drunks were starting to push and shove, so I started backing up into the hallway. Just as the drunks make a lunge towards me and I was about to defend myself, two strong arms grabbed me from behind and pinned my arms so I could not throw a punch. It was one of the other bouncers, and he was holding me yelling, 'No fighting, no fighting'. The problem was, I was copping a flogging from the front by the drunks because the idiot bouncer was stopping me from defending myself. This particular bouncer thought he was doing me a favour by stopping me from fighting.

So I had to push back through the inside door, hoping that someone would close the door while I got this idiot off my back. The door slammed behind me and what was left outside was a couple of aggressive drunks who could sort it out with the police. Needless to say, I was not too keen to work with him again.

He did not last long.

Robert

I was always happy to work with Robert. He started just after me, and was always plenty of fun. However, he had a bad temper and was much quicker to react and resort to throwing punches than I was.

On one night a brawl broke out inside the club and was spilling down the foyer stairs heading for the front door. I could see Robert in there and he was rolling on the ground, tussling with one of the regulars. The regular, who was quite a well-known model at the time, broke free and ran past me out the front door. Next thing Robert runs out after him and catches him just in front of the club. Robert had him by the throat and was forcing him down onto his knees. He was well out of control, screaming and swearing, intent on squeezing the life out of the model. So I walked over and calmly said to Robert that this was not such a good idea, and to let the poor guy go. In the meantime the other guy was passing out. Luckily Robert snapped out of it and let him go just in time, both of them collapsing in a heap in the gutter.

Doorman musing

Some nights were easy, nice and polite, while other nights were just war on the door. Many people would take it personally when they were denied entry because of their sad, alcohol-induced aggressive stupor. Many times my poor car got worked over because the drunk was too scared to confront the doorman. Or they would drive by and glare at you from a distance. The best was the threat that they were coming back with all their brothers and cousins to take on one usually cold and bored doorman who could not really give a damn how many brothers or cousins they were bringing back because he would just lock them out and call the police.

Working for nightclubs, the lines were always blurred. Who and where were the good guys? The manager of the club would get upset with me for letting in a couple of well-dressed transvestites, yet he would then usher through a couple of drug dealers packing weapons. I remember asking one well-dressed thug one night to show me his member pass, and he pulled back his coat to show me his Glock handgun. I looked up, and the manager quickly stepped in. 'He's okay,' he said.

Towards the end of my time on the door you needed a security license to work, and this was strictly policed by the licensing police who would just show up anytime to check you had a valid license. Quite often the drug dealers and the licensing police would be in the club at the same time. I always thought this a little strange.

From all my time working as a doorman/bouncer at several clubs, it was clear that alcohol and drugs dramatically change people. It always amazed me how someone could be your best friend when they wanted to come into the club, and then after a couple of drinks turn into your mortal enemy and try to remove your mouth from your face simply because you ask them to stop annoying a fellow patron.

Aggression and violence fuelled by booze and drugs put me at the coalface of learning about human nature and surviving in some pretty extreme situations. Clients would greet you at the beginning of the night like a long-lost brother, only to be turned into a vile aggressive creature full of anger and abuse by the end of the night, especially when you were trying to empty the premises at four in the morning after a long night.

It was on one such night that I asked the last man to leave and he refused several times, getting more and more aggressive each time I asked. Then he simply reached into his jacket, pulled out a gun, and placed it on the table in front of him. He then slurred that he was a copper and not going anywhere. I politely said, 'Let yourself out' and left the club, never to work in security again.

Chapter 4

Qantas 747 heading north

I was 24, living in Sydney's trendy inner west, running my own plumbing business, working as a doorman and teaching martial arts. I was independent, earning good money, and generally having a great time.

One hot Friday summer afternoon I was installing a corrugated iron roof on an old Federation house in the inner-city suburb of Leichhardt. Being fair skinned I was easily sunburned, and by the time 5pm came around I was hot, tired, and feeling the effects of the long day in the sun. I looked at my hands. They were cut to shreds by the sharp edges of the iron and black from the smears of silicone used to seal the roofing. When I first commenced plumbing, one of the old tradesman told me that I would cut, burn or take a lump out of my hand every day I worked as a plumber. He was right.

Just when I was thinking there had to be a better way to earn a living, exhausted, my gaze turned upwards towards the sound of roaring engines. I looked up and saw a magnificent sight: the underside of a Qantas 747

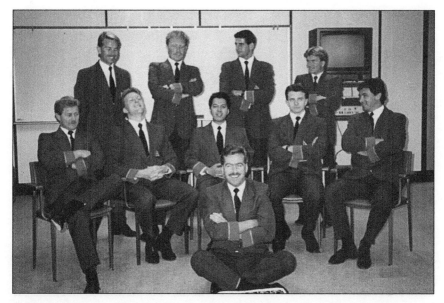

Initial training class with Qantas. I am in the middle row, second from the right.

heading north. As I watched the Jumbo disappear beyond the horizon, I was already making plans.

Six months later I was a Qantas Flight Attendant. The year was 1987. I was 24 years old and the world was at my fingertips. Working as a flight attendant enabled me to fly in and out of cities/countries and train on my downtime in locations that I chose. I signed up as a flight attendant so I could see the world and at the same time expand my martial arts knowledge and experience worldwide. I was ready for this, and the timing was perfect. This was really living my dream.

> *Recognise what makes you tick. I love the combat training in martial arts. Not because I like to fight, but because it brings out something deep and primal within me. To turn off or deny that part of me exists means I would not be able to express it in a positive and constructive way.*

Challenging myself

Wherever I could I would seek out new people to test myself. This was not out of anger or the desire to hurt people. The initial driving force was fuelled by the need to prove to myself that I was worth something as a human being. By training hard in martial arts and facing the fear of

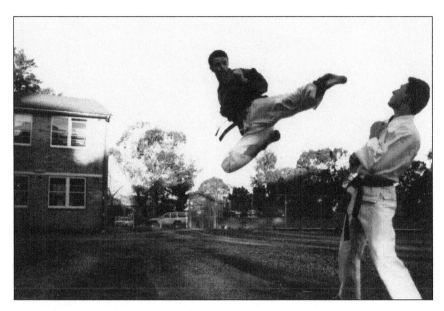

I am performing the flying side kick, an advanced kicking technique.

being hurt, injured or even killed, and not only surviving but flourishing, I started to believe in myself and my ability. I was training now to be the best I could be, and to reach my potential in sparring and more. Challenging myself to go further each time I accomplished a goal.

With the help of Qantas, I trained in America many times. I especially enjoyed training at the famous Dan Inosanto Academy (Dan Inosanto was a close friend and training partner of the late Bruce Lee). It was great because they had all kinds of lessons with world-class instructors. I picked up a lot of Thai kickboxing and Savate, a unique French approach to martial arts. I was lucky enough to train alongside Brandon Lee, son of Bruce Lee, who was a regular at Dan's classes. I found him to be quiet and polite, yet I could feel a deep sensitivity. I was shocked to hear of his early death in 1993.

Visiting and sparring at so many schools of martial arts all over the world, I soon learned not to judge anyone whatsoever. So many martial artists who were incredibly talented and pushed me to my limit had never trained outside of their own dojo, let alone trained and competed overseas.

Saturday mornings I would head down to Pico Boulevard in LA and spar with the students at Master Hee Ill Cho's taekwondo school. Master Hee

Ill Cho is famous for his incredible kicking skills, and is also a renowned author. Regardless of his great physical prowess, I found him to be aloof and unapproachable, and at times just plain grumpy. But he had a great team of trainers, and I will always remember one in particular. He matched me punch for punch and kick for kick, his defence was incredible, and I found myself on the back foot a lot. I don't remember his name, but he was one of the many who took me by surprise. It was always very humbling to train and spar with martial arts students who were only interested in sharpening their skills for personal growth and not for competition.

During one stay in LA I was invited to train with Joey Escobar. Joey was a top-ranked US karate champion who went on to captain the US karate team. I was pretty fit, as I was on my way to my first World Ju Jitsu Championship in North Carolina in 1990. The sparring was great, and I enjoyed the challenge of taking on one of America's top competitors, which was totally the opposite of Saturday sparring at Hee Ill Cho's Academy. Joey was fast and hard, but to my surprise I held my own, opening him up with fast kick counter-attacks. He was polite, but I could see that I was more than he expected. I was beginning to understand that I could match it with world-class competitors.

Little John

When I started entering competitions as a heavyweight, the weight range for heavyweight was anything over 85kg. I weighed 88kg, and so was considered light for a heavyweight. Many of my early taekwondo fights were against fighters between 100 and 120kg. Now I think there is a super heavyweight category, which I think is a great idea.

There was one fighter by the name of John Rhodes. I luckily managed to avoid him, as he was a member of the Australian Taekwondo Union of which I was not a member. John was the Australian Heavyweight Champion.

He was a man mountain and fast. He had a punch that could break you into pieces. I arrived to compete in an event at the Homebush Bay Stadium. It was a championship being run by a new Korean Master on the scene, a man by the name of Tiger Kim. I checked the draw to see who was fighting, and my heart skipped a beat when I saw that John was fighting. If I won my first fight, I would then meet him. I was scared, and I

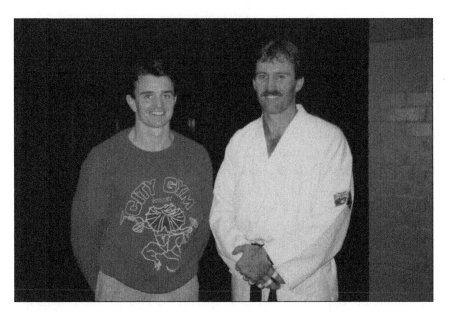

With Master John Rhodes on the right. A fierce competitor and champion.

wanted to pull out. But the moment I accepted that I did not need to win and to just let go, a calm resolve came over me. I easily won my first fight and met John in the final.

He smiled at me from across the other side of the ring, showing no front teeth. I was no longer scared. Destiny had played its hand. We circled each other, feeling each other out. I took the initiative and closed the distance. He hit me immediately in the chest with a right punch that knocked me back. It was a crushing blow, and it reverberated throughout my entire body. I continued and fought hard, and even scored some clean hits, but his experience was the telling factor and he won. I earned his respect, which was an honour.

After the match, John invited me to come and train with him at his studio, as he was impressed with my skills. I trained with John for a number of months in my lead-up to my next training trip in Korea. John even let on to me that I had hurt him in our fight. Naturally he did not show it. John was a good man, and he has my respect.

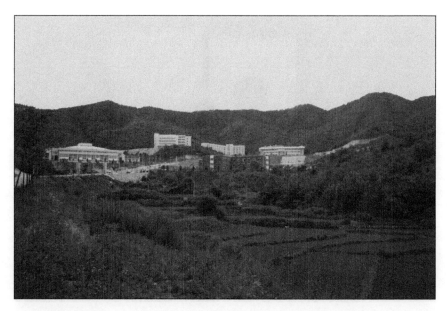

Yudo College situated on the side of a mountain at Yong In, approximately one hour from Seoul, South Korea.

Crazy Korea, 1989

Taekwondo has played a large part in my development as a martial artist. My first taekwondo instructor, Master Tim Hassall, was very progressive, and we cross-trained a lot in boxing and kickboxing. Back in 1980, when I started taekwondo, kickboxing was getting popular, and was a huge innovation to traditional martial arts.

In 1989, one of my students and I got the opportunity to train in taekwondo in the place that it originated – South Korea. We travelled to a small country town near Seoul called Yong-In. Yong-In is home to the famous Yudo College that went on to become Yong-In University – a private university that sits on the side of a mountain. Students at Yudo College can take a four-year degree in physical education majoring in taekwondo or judo. For the next two weeks, I would fully immerse myself and train in taekwondo with the Korean team.

I really did not know what I was getting myself into. All I knew was that people who trained at Yudo College never feared being kicked ever again. I was not scared, I was terrified. But I knew I had to do this. I was ready for the challenge, as all my training up until now had prepared me for this.

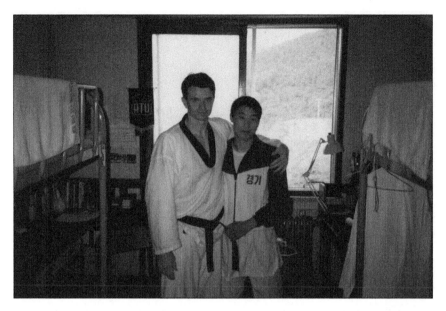

After many rounds of tough sparring, friends were made. In the small dorm at Yudo College.

The college itself was old and run down, but the water was clean and the air fresh, and the food was basically just the traditional Korean dish of Kimchi and rice. The accommodation was in small dormitories, bunking in with the Korean students. This really was total immersion.

The first training session of the day started at 6am and went for 90 minutes. We ran and ran and ran, up and down the road to nowhere that went straight up into the mountain. It did not go anywhere, and was built purely for fitness and conditioning. I've always enjoyed running hills, as it is essential for kicking power. But I was struggling with the piggybacks and jump squats, and I was determined not to bring up the dinner from the night before.

At 11am the main session of the day started with a frenzy of kicks and pain. Fifty very passionate Korean fighters, two brave Aussies, and the coach Master Ko (ex-World Heavyweight Taekwondo Champion) who walked around the huge modern studio with a bamboo cane. My training partner that I went with only lasted the first training session. I don't blame him. It was brutal and tough.

The toughest fights for me were against the Korean taekwondo fighters at Yudo College, South Korea. I had to play their game though.

For the next two weeks the Korean fighters threw every possible attack at me, lining up one after the other to fight and beat me down. Though I was out on my feet many times, I never dropped to one knee. I constantly endured the onslaught, and it was ferocious. We trained together and lived in close quarters for the entire time.

I remember an American team that arrived to train about a week into my stay. They were loud and very nervous. During their first sparring session, the Koreans rushed to partner with the Americans. By this stage they were not so keen to fight me as I was starting to bang them up a little.

The fighting rounds started, and the Koreans launched themselves full force into the Americans. Within a blink of an eye the American team was littered across the floor. I was astounded. I had been copping the might of the Korean team for a week now, and here was a top American team downed in the first 10 seconds. To top it all off, in the first training session a week before I slipped on the floor and tore a groin muscle. I could not even raise a knee I was in so much pain.

The two weeks soon passed. On the last day, it was my last training session and the Korean team captain huddled his team together. This was no small team – it numbered over 50. They had an hour to break me.

One after the other they came at me. I had nothing to lose. I smashed my fists into whatever came close – arms, chests and, if I could cheat, faces. I unleashed full force. The captain was screaming to every fighter that I faced.

The last fighter finally got me. I felt his kick across the side of my face and wobbled. As I vainly fought to regain my legs, he spun and caught me with a full back kick knocking the wind out of me. Still, I was not going down. I stumbled to the side desperately trying to breathe, at the same time waiting for the last killer blow. I remained standing as the round finished.

I walked off the mat with a great sense of accomplishment. I climbed the Everest of martial arts again. I left there proud that I had survived, and I never feared a kick ever again.

There is a certain mindset and way of thinking that has enabled me to survive, endure and ultimately excel, breaking through incredible physical and emotional barriers. I use this simple philosophy: When you think you have had enough, it is only a thought. You may be capable of so much more. You do not have to believe the thoughts, but if you do they can either empower you or defeat you. You choose. I learned to just acknowledge the thoughts, then keep moving in the direction I am going in.

Surprise in Thailand

The year was 1989, and I was recently back from my time in South Korea. I was working on the way to London and happened to have a short stopover in Bangkok. I was walking near the hotel and just happened to stumble across the Thailand Taekwondo Headquarters. I was surprised, as I had walked the same way many times before and had never noticed it. Curious, I thought I would take a look inside.

The studio (or *dojang* in Korean) was back off the street in an old warehouse. Thinking back now, I am amazed that I actually stumbled onto the place. Inside there was a small area for training and a separate competition area that was just a large warehouse space with a wooden floor and a competition square taped out for a ring. This place oozed intensity. The Thais are famous for their fighting ferocity, and I could feel that this was a serious place.

There was a poster on the front door advertising their Annual Thailand Championships coming up in a couple of weeks. It just so happened that I would be passing through Bangkok again on that exact day. The thought crossed my mind that it would be great to enter the competition, but being accepted to compete would be a long shot.

Just when I was about to leave, the dojang (studio) manager came out of her office to say hello. She was so friendly, and even invited my mate Steve and I in for tea. I told her of my martial arts experience and my time in Korea, and mentioned that I would be in Bangkok in two weeks and asked would it be okay if I came to watch the championship. She was really excited and straight away offered me a chance to compete, which I readily accepted. I guess they didn't get many foreigners wanting to compete in those days. I was pretty confident and a little smug, thinking it would be a breeze as you don't see many big Thais.

A foolish thought, as I was to learn.

I spent the next two weeks training my heart out. The only thing I could not prepare for was the Bangkok heat and humidity, so I knew I had to be fit. If you are not fit you lose, and it makes any fight a long, hard grind. I have learned my lesson fighting when I have not been fit, and I made a promise to myself never to do it again. This competition was three rounds of three minutes, which is a long fight. So I knew I had to be in the best shape of my life.

On a hot, steamy Sunday morning Steve, who was to be my corner man, and I arrived at the Thai Taekwondo Headquarters. I was positive and ready, but naturally a little apprehensive as I was unsure how this would go. The dojang was a frenzy of movement with numerous competitors readying for action. The ring was simply a square marked on the large timber floor, and there was a small grandstand that was filling fast. I still had not seen anyone who resembled my size, and upon asking about my fight I was politely told to kindly wait. So wait I did.

The smells from the busy Bangkok streets were overpowered by the smell of combat. The instant I smelled the sharpness of the Tiger Balm my stomach twinged with fear. The self-talk began, and it was the beginning of my battle.

Maybe I won't have to fight. That would be okay. No-one would mind. This is crazy. You made it this far, that's enough. It's too dangerous. These were just a few thoughts that started. But I knew this was normal. I acknowledged the thoughts and kept on with my preparation regardless.

The thing is, fight or flight is a natural response to fear and stress and you cannot suppress it. So I would let my mind chatter away and just let my body move regardless. I learned to trust my body, as though it had a mind of its own and knew best.

The fights started in a wild frenzy of legs, arms and violence. I was astounded at the quality of the competitors. The large crowd vied for the best position, and were packed right up to the edge of the ring. The atmosphere was serious, but you could not get over the fact that the Thais were really enjoying themselves. There was this feeling of infectious joy.

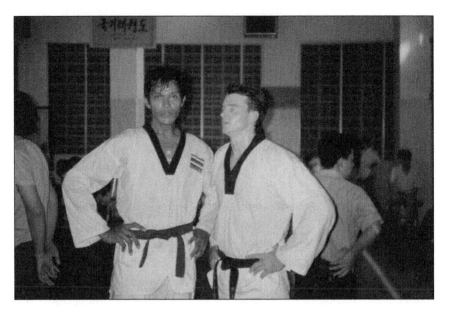

Me after fighting Middleweight champion Montien.

Now taekwondo may have been my first martial art, but there were two distinct styles. The traditional style I trained in, and the competition style that has gone on to become an Olympic sport. The styles could have easily been two completely different martial arts altogether. As my style of martial arts developed I wanted to teach a system of fighting that covered all ranges of combat – kicking and punching, close-quarter combat, grappling, throwing and ground defence. Taken as a whole it has developed into a formidable system. But even better, it can be broken into its individual components, allowing you to train in any system anywhere in the world and hold your own. You don't need to be an expert. You just need to know enough to enjoy the experience.

This is what I was doing on a balmy day in Bangkok: putting my theory and the system to the test. I was not a great taekwondo competitor, but I wanted to see if I could at least hold my own.

Montien was at least six inches taller than me. Though he was lighter, I could see that he was fit and strong. He was a member of the Thailand Taekwondo Team. I had never seen a Thai that tall before. Apparently he was a model and popular on TV commercials. It was not hard to see that he was their hero, as he was greeted like a celebrity. It was at about this time I started to get nervous and seriously wonder what I had gotten myself into.

We were the last fight of the day, and it had been a long day. I was not sure how much of my strength and fitness had been sapped out of me through the heat and nervous energy. When preparing for a competition, it is not just the fight that you prepare for. You need to take into account the energy used up through nerves and anticipation. I have seen so many competitors who have not taken this into account and found themselves exhausted before the fight even commences.

Steve helped me put on the thin body protection and headgear. No gloves, foot pads or shin protectors. Just the way I like it. He was stoic and quiet. Steve and I became mates the moment we met at flight attendant school, and we have remained great mates through thick and thin now for 30 years. We still laugh about this day: the two Aussie boys way out of their league and the only non-Thai people in the building. He enjoyed it so much he later nicknamed me 'The Bangkok Bomber'.

It was time. As I stood on the edge of the ring the feeling was similar to a surfer on the tip of a huge wave, just about to take off: fear and exhilaration, taunting death. Steve reassured me with a pat on the back and simply said, 'You'll be right mate'.

Montien was fast and dangerous. This was his house, and the crowd were loving every minute. He came at me immediately, looking to finish the fight early. He blasted a hard, turning kick to my body from the start that really hurt. I was way out of my depth, but I was in it now. He threw everything at me in the first round, wave after wave. One false move by me, one misjudged technique, and it would surely be an ambulance ride for me.

The second round started with pretty much the same intensity as the first. But I was starting to find my mark and hit him. I was hitting him with all my power, and by the end of the round I could see he was starting to hesitate. The third round he was tiring, and I was getting stronger. But I still could not risk a lapse in concentration.

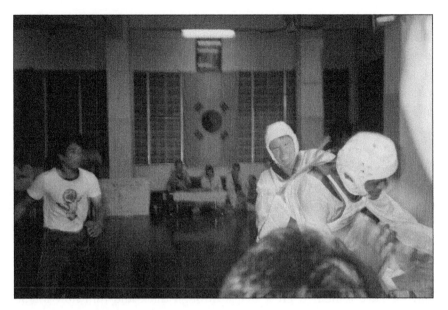

Intensely chasing Montien into the crowd.

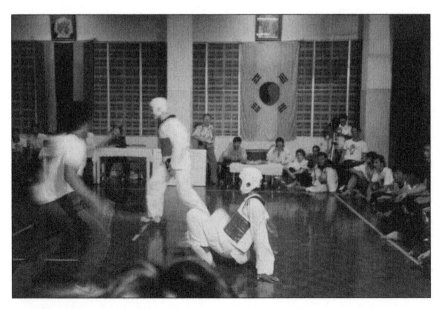

Knocking Montien down in the third round.

Late in the round my kick found his chin and down he went. He was up quickly, but I could see it was over for him. I continued to stalk him, and even teased him a little. By the end of the fight we were both exhausted, so we sat as we waited for the decision. I was pretty sure that if I did not knock him out I was going to lose. But I didn't mind either way. The entire experience was exhilarating. I was over the moon that I had experienced this and survived.

We were marshalled into the centre of the ring to find out who had won. I got the shock of my life when both our arms were raised as winners. It was a very kind gesture of sportsmanship, and indicative of the kind and humble nature of the Thai people. My knuckles and shins were bloodied, battered and bruised. I put my arm around my mate Steve and we made our way limping to a waiting tuk tuk. It had been a great experience, and we were looking forward to reliving it over a couple of cold beers.

> *Only when you accept that fear is part of the process – feel it, see it, observe it – then quickly move on, not allowing the fear to kneejerk you backward towards habitual patterns of fear, and you strengthen the courage around fear, will you slowly 'power up' your life as boundaries that have restricted you crumble.*

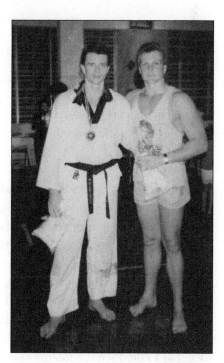

Battered and bloodied after the fight. With my mate from the Qantas Crew, Steve.

Chapter 5

Life and death at Crown St Sydney, 1990

B y now I had been studying martial arts for 10 years or more. I was a 2nd Dan Black Belt (levels of black belt go up in grades called dans) in taekwondo, had ample experience in ju jitsu, was competing regularly, and working security on nightclub doors. All in all, I was in pretty good shape.

It was about 7pm, and my girlfriend at the time and I had just finished training at City Gym on Crown St and were heading back to the car. It was a normal day, nothing out of the ordinary, and this had been a regular routine for many months. My girlfriend was getting into the passenger side of the car as I was getting into the driver's side. Out of the shadows a figure went straight up to my girlfriend and demanded money. I could not really see what was going on as I was halfway into the car. Next thing you know there is another man walking around the car towards me. It was dark already, so it was hard to see what he was like. I knew something was wrong as I could see the intention in his eyes.

He said to me, 'Give me your money or we will stab your friend'. (Or other more graphic words to that effect.) She screamed at me that the guy close to her had a knife. As the second man walked around the car to me, I yelled at her to get into the car and lock the door. She hesitated, so I let it be known quite clearly what she had to do.

She jumped in the car and locked the door as the man closest to her hammered the top of the car with the butt of his knife. A second later the man closest to me lunged at my chest with a long blade. I was fast enough to just pull away as he took a second swing at me, catching me on my sleeve and ripping my hoodie. Luckily it did not bite the skin of my arm. I immediately made distance between me and the two men. But they saw me as an easy target and quickly followed, which was okay as it allowed my girlfriend time to get away in the car.

As we rounded a corner onto Crown St, opposite what used to be the Hard Rock Café, I kept talking. 'You don't need the knife,' I said. 'You could take me without it. Just put the knife down and I will give you what you want.'

The first man put his knife down on the footpath and, to my astonishment, pulled his arm back to punch me in the head. I moved very quickly, maintaining balance and putting years of martial arts training into action. Striking hard and fast, my weapons found their mark, easily taking out the first man. He fell at my feet and tried to grab my leg. I continued to strike hard, and he let go. The second man saw what was coming and made a very hasty retreat.

This was a very ugly experience. It took very clear thinking and presence to be able to hold it together and respond effectively. If I had not had years of martial arts training, the outcome could have been so much different. How many stories do we read or hear that someone somewhere has been stabbed and killed?

Even knife experts get stabbed, Manila, 1990

After being attacked by the knife-wielding thugs in Sydney, I felt a deep sense of vulnerability that I had not felt for many years. After all my years of learning how to kick and punch, the main thought that came to me as I was preparing to defend myself was to keep both feet firmly on the ground and do not kick. The slightest error in judgement could have had me losing my balance, which could have been lethal. So with this new-found information I was determined to learn about knives and knife defence.

The knife gives anyone incredible power, as you do not need to be able to fight or spend years learning martial arts to use one. A knife in the hands of someone intent on using it becomes a lethal weapon, and as I was soon to learn even with extensive knife defence training there are no guarantees.

Through my contacts at the local martial arts supplies I was given the number of Ray Floro. I trained with Ray, and soon came to respect his ability as a knife practitioner. It just so happened that I had a work trip to Manila coming up, so Ray put me in contact with one of his teachers, Rommie Macapacal.

The first time I met Rommie was in the car park of my hotel in Manila. Rommie was shortish but very powerfully built. His forearms were huge, no doubt from years of training with knives, sticks and his weapon of choice, the Filipino machete.

Speaking with Rommie for the first time, I quickly summed up that you would not want to get on the bad side of a knife fighter here in Manila. Rommie showed me the set of sharpened machetes he kept in his car – a necessity, as he recently issued a challenge match to another fighter for slighting his reputation. He was serious, and went on to explain that you cannot back away from a challenge as his family's and system's reputation would be on the line. Though at the time I could not understand this way of thinking, it is a concept I was going to come to understand more when I started to develop my own systems of training and teaching.

As I was staying in Manila for five days (the first of many trips to Manila to train), Rommie picked me up and told me we were going straight to his master's place to introduce me and to train. We were going to meet the famous grandmaster of Filipino fighting arts, Antonio Illustrisimo (or Tatang as he is affectionately known). We made our way deep into the slums of Manila to where Tatang, aged in his late 80s, lived with his much younger wife.

The slum was full of life – barefoot kids kicking balls and splashing in dirty puddles, scrawny dogs barking at us as we passed. And the smell reminded me of the slums in India. (You never forget that smell.)

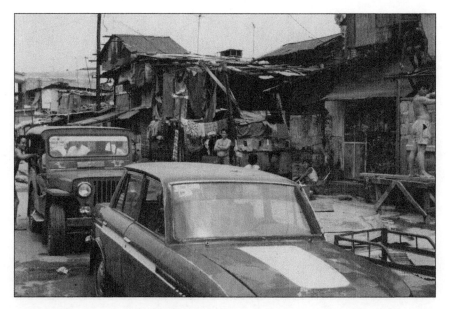

Tatang's home in the Manila slums. We spent many hours training there.

I ducked my head and entered a small shack. The roof was simple corrugated iron and the floor was packed dirt. The table and chairs had been moved to the side to make a small space to train. This simple hut was now the world headquarters of the Illustrisimo Eskrima Academy. I have come to believe over all my years of travelling and training that it is not where you set up your academy that matters. It is the strength of the heart that pumps within it.

Rommie introduced me to Tatang, who warmly greeted me. I was also introduced to Tony Diego, another of Tatang's top students and, like Rommie, lethal. We briefly sat and chatted, eating plain salted crackers and drinking warm Fanta.

The training started almost immediately, with Tony feeding Tatang a full range of attacks with the short stick. Tatang was fast and efficient, smothering and countering Tony's every move. They switched between knife, stick and machete, and the fundamentals were the same for each weapon. The Illustrismo system is a combat-based system that flows and counters. The moves are designed to take your opponent out as fast as possible. The three men –Tony, Rommie and Tatang – switched between each other, and for 30 minutes put on one of the most memorable displays

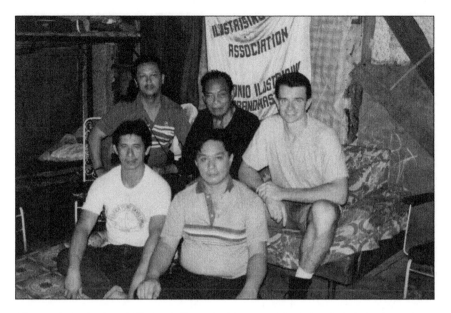

Tatang sitting in the middle back. Rommie Macapagal is sitting directly in front of me, with Tony Diego next to him.

of martial arts prowess I have ever witnessed. But the most amazing thing about this display was that Tatang was technically blind.

I started my first session with Tony Diego under the watchful eye of Rommie and Tatang. In between the odd rat the size of a cat running through the middle of the room, we worked the knife against knife, machete and stick defence, which was all great training. The defensive angles and cuts were lethal, and I quickly realised that with even only a little of this training, if I had a knife in a defensive situation I could quite easily cut my opponent to shreds.

The problem was I did not want to carry a knife with me at home back in Australia. So we practiced empty hand defence against a knife. Now these masters were the best around, and had all been in knife fights, but as Rommie said, 'It does not matter how good you are with a knife. You are always going to get cut. It is just a matter of where and how bad'. Even a knife in the hands of an untrained partner is a deadly weapon. They all had the scars to show from being cut in knife fights.

Satisfied with my research and training with knives, I now realised I survived the knife attack in Sydney by using great communication and remaining calm, and felt happy. The simple skills I learned in Manila were fun and effective, but I still think the best defence is to avoid all confrontation no matter what. You will never see the knife. You will only feel it. I continued to meet and train with Tatang, Tony and Rommie whenever I was in Manila. Tatang passed away in 1997, and the association was split up amongst his senior students. My mate Ray Floro continues to teach his own system of martial arts worldwide.

The Guardian Angels, USA, 1990

My quest to test my system took me to some rather strange locations and situations. Back in the late 80s and early 90s there was a group of vigilantes that was getting quite a lot of media attention. Founded by Curtis Sliwa, the Guardian Angels claimed to take up the slack where regular law enforcement let the public down. Their thing was simply presence and observation. If there were drug dealers in a certain location, the Guardian Angels would simply go and hang out in the same areas and without violence persuade them to move on. In principle it all sounded really good, but the presence of the Guardian Angels upset a lot of organised crime and, funnily enough, regular law enforcement. The regular law enforcement looked at the Angels as a danger to themselves and not properly trained. There was also the often-blurred line between the police and criminals, and the public they were supposed to be protecting.

The group was well organised. They had chapters in most cities in the USA, as well as in Canada and several European countries. And they were making a difference. My first experience with the Angels was in LA. This would be a dangerous yet eye-opening experience.

As I write this many years later, I'm trying to revisit the mindset that drove me to want to expose myself to potentially life-threatening situations. Why was I constantly seeking to pressure-test my martial arts skills? I think that initially I wanted to prove to myself that I could face my fears that had accumulated over the years, and not have them cripple me. Each time I did this it set the bar a little higher, and I would seek out more intense and dangerous experiences.

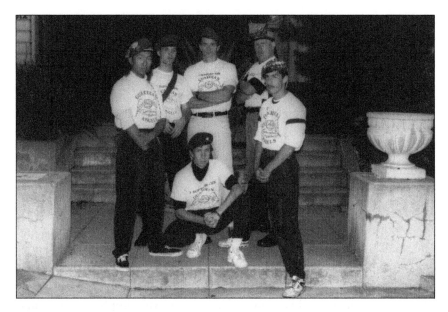

Going out on patrol with the Guardian Angels in Hollywood LA, USA. I am standing in the back middle.

Training in the dojo, or competing in competitions, was always against trained fighters. So although the sparring was often a torrid affair, the movements were in a way predictable. I wanted to prove to myself that I could cope with anything, no matter how hard or unexpected. I approached the group to see if I could patrol with them.

I was in LA a lot with my other job as a flight attendant, and would duck away at night to patrol the seedy streets of West Hollywood. Highly risky, and I could have lost my job if anyone found out. This is the first time I have shared this with anyone.

The LA chapter had about 30 Angels at various levels. The patrols consisted of 8-10 people, mostly ex-gang members or people genuinely wanting to help make the streets a little safer. Knowing that the situation on patrol could go pear-shaped in a blink of an eye, the fear of doing something so potentially dangerous was there from the moment I put on the Guardian Angel t-shirt and beret.

The first session was a weekly training session where you learned the skills of how to cope with the various scenarios that would happen on the street.

These training sessions were more about survival, and I really got to test my fighting skills against the other men in the team. Most were from street gangs, and had learned enough about dirty fighting to survive most encounters. But my basic martial arts skills certainly came in handy as the drills often turned violent. In LA, we spent the nights chasing crack dealers and gang members off the streets. I thought it was all a bit too quiet, but was assured by the other team members that it could all go very wrong at any time.

I was 27, and in North Carolina USA for the World Ju Jitsu Championships in 1990. So I thought I would fly over to Manhattan, New York, to try my luck with the New York chapter of the Guardian Angels. The New York team met early in the evening in a dingy room on Times Square that looked like it housed the homeless. There I met Curtis and his then wife. It was all very pleasant and I was welcomed with open arms. I was surprised by how casual it was. We quickly split into groups.

As we headed out on patrol I was looking around, wondering what I had gotten myself into. They were an interesting mix of white collar business types, African-Americans, Latinos, ex-gang members and regular citizens wanting to make a difference. All were keen to get out onto the streets.

Our aim on this night was to be a presence around a couple of street corners that are used for prostitution and drug dealing. This was the way they worked. They would just stand near where the prostitutes worked, and by their presence clients would be hesitant to approach. This would have a significant effect on their ability to make money. The intention was to have them move on and work somewhere else. But on this night it was all going to backfire.

We partnered up and started walking to near where they were working. My partner was a wiry Hispanic ex-gang member who joined the Angels after he lost his brother to gang violence. He told me to stay close and not to say anything, probably nervous at having someone so new as a partner. I did not blame him for being nervous. I was a white middle-class man walking into some of the most violent streets in New York, looking for trouble.

As they saw us approaching, the prostitutes started to yell and abuse us, and it looked like it was going to get violent very quickly. We backed off to another street corner and waited for things to calm down.

The police were on the scene very quickly, pulling up in front of us in a typical New York fashion, sirens blaring, tyres screeching. I was amazed at how quickly they arrived. Two very large and not-so-friendly patrol officers jumped out of the car and demanded to know why we were harassing the prostitutes. This was a complex situation as I can only wonder why these New York Police officers were protecting the prostitutes. I think it was a mixture of the Guardian Angels getting in the way of the police and a behind-the-scenes agreement between the prostitutes and the police.

Either way, I felt it was a very dangerous and highly volatile situation. They made us sit down cross-legged in one line, backs against the wall, and asked to see some identification. The head of our team was off to the side in a heated discussion with one of the officers.

We were very close to being arrested. And I know from talking with the Angels that you were not welcome in any police lockup if you were wearing a Guardian Angel beret and shirt. We sat for ages and just waited. I was scared and way out of my comfort zone.

In the end, the prostitute who was doing all the screaming got into the back of one of the patrol cars and drove away with the police. We were allowed to go, but threatened with arrest if we did not move on. The whole incident was very ugly and very wrong. It was obvious that the Guardian Angels were not a welcome presence on the streets, with both the criminals and the police taking action against them. It was a close call, and I realised this was not a good way to spend my holiday.

World Championships, North Carolina, 1990

The first world championship I competed in was in 1990 in North Carolina, USA. At 27 I was selected to be on the Australian Ju Jitsu team after winning the Australian Championships on the Gold Coast. To prepare, I trained for a month in Japan, so I was pretty fit and ready to compete. As this was the main selection for the Australian team, the fights were intense. I ended up winning 12 fights and drawing one.

The drawn fight was quite controversial. I never missed with my front leg, high turning kick. I'd honed and sharpened it to perfection. In my first bout I landed the kick immediately, scoring a clean point as it hit the side

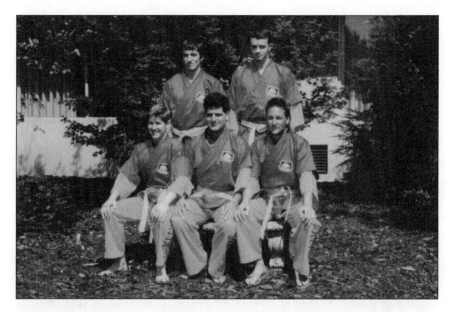

The Australian Ju Jitsu team competing in the World Championships in North Carolina 1990.

of my opponent's head. But he went down, claiming I had struck him on the side of his neck – an illegal technique. Believe me, if I had kicked him in the side of the neck it would not have been by accident.

He wallowed on the ground for a couple of minutes while he recovered. It was embarrassing to watch. Due to his convincing dive, he was awarded a point for my so-called illegal technique. As he was now one point ahead, he tried to protect his lead by defending and moving away from me. I scored a late point, drawing the bout. I went on to win my next 12 fights to become the overall Australian Ju Jitsu Champion, and was chosen for the Australian Team.

At the championship in North Carolina the format of the fighting was point fighting, so it really suited the sharp shooters who were quickly in and out, scoring points then retreating. This style of fighting does not flow, so it is hard to put combinations together. Regardless, it was fun as I got to have several fights, winning some and losing some.

I beat the Puerto Rican and Costa Rican fighters, then went on to fight the USA fighter. It was a tough win. His name was Warren Owsley, and he would go on to become World Champion in the years to come. He sadly passed away in 2015.

I then came up against the current World Heavyweight champion from Canada, Sean Stewart. That was a huge learning experience. He soundly beat me, and I respected him even more as he did not hurt me in the process. A true champion.

At the time, the Australian Ju Jitsu Team was run by one of Australia's leading and most respected ju jitsu masters. After the world championships he was arrested on numerous counts of child molestation and sent to prison for five years. I was totally shocked, but it wasn't the first or the last time that so-called martial arts masters were found to be breaking the law.

> *Combat. Start from stillness. Be neutral. Don't give your opponent a chance to form an opinion. No show of external. Act quickly and immediately. While they are thinking, you are responding. Stick to basics. Learn them well. Maintain balance. Lose it and you lose. Strike hard and quickly. Maintain form. Maintain constant awareness. Turn on, switch off, move on. Finish with stillness.*

The birth of mixed martial arts

After getting my black belt in taekwondo, even though I was trained well in stand-up fighting including boxing and kickboxing I felt there was a real flaw in my training. If someone grabbed me I could easily be thrown, and I was a quick target if fighting on the ground. So I set about finding a good ju jitsu school.

Ju jitsu was hard to find back then (1984). There was no Brazilian Ju Jitsu (BJJ) or mixed martial arts (MMA), and about the closest you could get to finding a good grappling school was judo.

By chance I stumbled on a very traditional ju jitsu dojo in Sydney called Tenjin-Shin-yo Ryu Ju Jitsu close to where I was living. Tenjin Shin-yo Ryu was one of the original styles that judo founder Jigaro Kano studied before he founded judo. So I was lucky enough to start training at Tenjin. At the same time I also started with the Sydney University Judo Club. I eventually went to Japan and was graded to black belt in Tenjin Shin-yo Ryu in 1989.

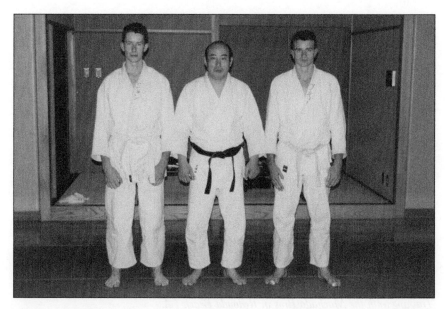

Me in Tokyo, Japan training with Tenjin Shinyo Ryu Ju Jitsu headmaster Kubota Sensei and my brother John.

The judo training was fantastic, and great to combine with my stand-up fighting skills. The more judo I learned, the more I started to apply the grappling and ground fighting in free sparring, together with kicks and punches. This new style of sparring that included kicking and punching, throwing and ground fighting was unheard of in the middle to late 80s, and I was fascinated by the prospect of increasing my skills and having the advantage over other fighters.

> *When a boxer punches you kick, when a kicker kicks you grapple. The master hones the ability to recognise the threat and counter into the gaps.*

I trained with the University Judo Team for five years. My sound basics of judo went on to form a large part of the ground defensive moves that I would later teach. I still believe that the basic ground positions you learn in judo are fundamental in being able to take control on the ground.

It was through a martial arts magazine that I saw an advertisement for a video that highlighted another form of ju jitsu that was taking on and beating all challengers. This was Gracie Ju Jitsu, and the style they did was Brazilian Ju Jitsu (BJJ). This was 1988. Months later I found myself in LA,

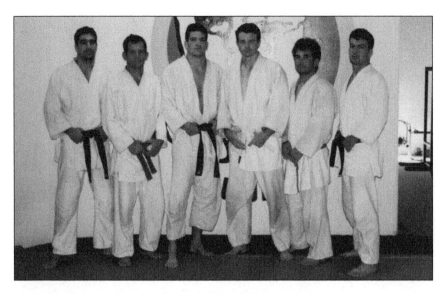

Training with the Machado Bros in Redondo Beach LA.

USA heading towards the house of Rorian Gracie, the son of the great Helio Gracie, brother to Royce and Rickson Gracie, and founder of the Ultimate Fighting Challenge (UFC).

The Gracie family had not been in LA very long. Rorian invited me into his house, a plain fibro house in the suburbs of Torrance, and made me very welcome. The garage attached to the house was converted into a studio, and there were students coming in and out. I purchased the video I had seen in the magazine from Rorian himself.

Little did I know that the Gracies would pioneer the explosion of BJJ worldwide and start the famous UFC. I trained at the Gracie Ju Jitsu studio in Torrance, California whenever I could make it. I had the pleasure of doing a quick round of wrestling with the great Rickson Gracie, which was over very quickly. Wrestling Rickson, he easily manipulated me and had an answer for all of my moves. He was graceful and ruthless at the same time, exploiting my weaknesses and playing with me like a cat plays with a mouse. It was great for experience, and all good knowledge that I would use to help steer me towards the development of my own martial arts system in the future. I continued to train in BJJ and judo, and started to train with the Machado Brothers, cousins of the Gracie family, in BJJ whenever I was in LA for work.

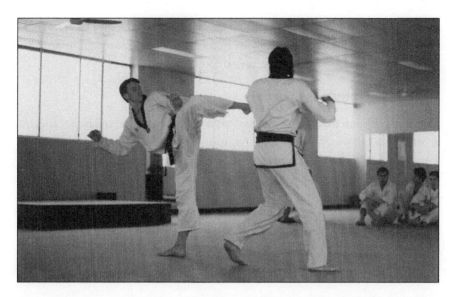

Sparring Big Col Handley, nine times Australian Heavyweight Taekwondo Champion.

The greatest accomplishment in martial arts is to be able to slice through life uninterrupted, smoothly, gracefully, having just as much success and failure as everyone else, but being totally unaffected as you ride the highs and the lows.

Training in Sydney

When I was 28, I was training and sparring several times a week and competing once every three weeks. But although I am very competitive by nature, I never really got into martial arts tournaments. I enjoyed the training in the lead-up, but was never aggressive enough to want to pursue a career in competitive fighting. Although I won a lot of my fights and was thrilled at the time, the good winning feelings would never last. My training partners included Adam Watt (four-times World Kickboxing Champion and Commonwealth Boxing Champion), Colin Handley (nine-times Australian Taekwondo Champion), Rob Mataic, a mate who I stood toe to toe with on many occasions, as well as several other well-known fighters at the time. We were all good mates, but regardless we all wanted to win. The sparring was thrilling and hard, and we often walked within a razor's edge of injury. One false move equalled injury for weeks – or worse.

Col Handley was well known for his axe kick and chest-crushing punch. He sent Dimi Tops to hospital for a week or so after he started having heart problems following a chest punch.

If you choose non-violence, it is good to have the backup of a good robust martial art. True non-violence is something you evolve into as the desire to win is replaced by a softer form of martial arts that is kinder to the body.

Deeper yearnings

I enjoyed the intensity of training, and it was great to be in shape. But no matter how fit I was, how good my techniques were, how many competitions I won or how many different sparring partners I experienced, there was an emptiness in what I was doing, and a feeling there had to be more to it. There was no doubt that the martial arts were a test of spirit. But when I was 17 my original desire was to find a true master who could guide and mentor my martial arts journey. Over the decade since then that desire had been lost, with me realising it was because of my fixation to be the best and the strongest in an effort to come to terms with my deeper insecurities.

From my experience in martial arts to that point, I felt there were so many different versions and interpretations of what martial arts really represented. There was no one governing body, and very little government regulation. Anyone could strap on a black belt and open up a school. It was really hard to get a foothold on what and who was real, and what was not. I met so many wankers, and their martial arts were nothing more than a temple made of paper cards.

Luckily there was a deeper yearning developing within me – a need to find more substance to the martial arts and meaning to life. The harder I tried to ignore this pull, the more it kept coming up. I knew that I did want to continue my martial arts journey, but was unsure how this would fit in with my quest for a deeper understanding of life.

So I started to push harder to try and find out whether martial arts were all physical, or whether they could serve as a vehicle to understand the body, mind and spirit and eventually lead to self-knowledge.

Use the dojo as a place to become still and neutral. Once you step onto the mat, release into the present moment and leave all else behind. Whether it is sparring or normal class, your attitude and focus should be the same: still and neutral, ready to respond.

Chapter 6
Daito Ryu Aiki ju jitsu

Back in 1987, I happened to see a very small video clip of a martial arts demonstration filmed in Japan. And I was mesmerised by what I saw – the swiftness of movement, the precision of the lethal techniques. I had to find more information.

In 1980s Australia, little was known about Daito Ryu Aiki ju jitsu. Even in Japan it has long been considered a relic of a pre-war era, at best the poor cousin of its modern-day cognate Aikido. But nothing could be further from the truth.

Daito Ryu has always been a conservative and somewhat secretive martial art. Its most famous exponent, Takeda Sokaku, only ever taught people of high social standing such as politicians, teachers, police and military people. Before that, the art belonged exclusively to the Aizu clan in Japan, and was never allowed to be shown to outsiders.

Takeda Sokaku was probably one of the last true warriors. At the turn of the 19th century he spent his time roaming Japan, taking on challengers and perfecting his sword and ju jitsu techniques against anyone foolish

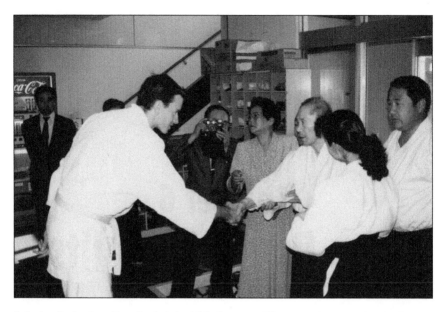

Meeting Daito Ryu Founder Sokaku Takeda's son Tokimune, who succeeded the founder. An auspicious occasion.

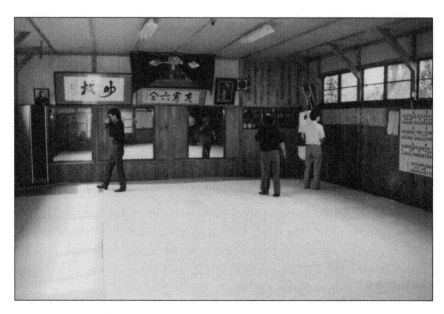

The Daitokan in Abashiri Hokkaido Japan, the world headquarters of Daito Ryu Aiki Ju Jitsu. It has since been demolished.

enough to take him on. Although only 5ft tall he was feared and respected as a great martial artist, and continued to travel around Japan teaching and spreading Daito Ryu well into his eighties.

Takeda's most famous student was Morihei Ueshiba, the founder of modern-day Aikido. In fact, without Takeda Sensei's teachings Aikido in its present form would probably never exist today. Ueshiba Sensei studied the art from 1915 to 1937, and received instructor's certification in the art (Kyoju Dairi) and also the *Goshin'yo no te scroll*, which was the highest level of Daito Ryu awarded in those days.

Up until the beginning of the Second World War, Ueshiba Sensei actually taught Daito Ryu Aiki ju jitsu at his own dojo. Although it is true to say there are some vague similarities between Aikido and Daito Ryu (they both begin and end with courtesy and their final goal is the development of spirit, love and harmony), Ueshiba's Aikido is a much-weakened form of combat void of the original form.

Aikido, which is a purely defensive and spiritually orientated martial art, works on blending and harmonising with the opponent after he has initiated an attack. Whereas Sokaku's Aiki ju jitsu is a method of hand-to-hand combat primarily concerned with repelling an attack immediately, making ample use of strikes against anatomical weak points, joint dislocation, breaks, throws and chokes.

In 1987, although very small and hard to find, Daito Ryu Aiki ju jitsu had remained remarkably intact since Takeda Sokaku Sensei started disseminating the art throughout Japan. Periodically put on hold during the Second World War, the art in its original form was still very much alive in a small industrial suburb in the outskirts of Tokyo.

The Daito Ryu Aiki ju jitsu of the Shinbukan Dojo in Tokyo might very well have been one of the last martial art frontiers in the world to be untouched by commercialism and sensationalism. The dojo itself is on the third floor of Kondo Sensei's construction company.

The moment you laid eyes on the building, you got the idea there was something uniquely different about the contents of the building in front of you. Beside the entrance was a bronze moulded nameplate proudly

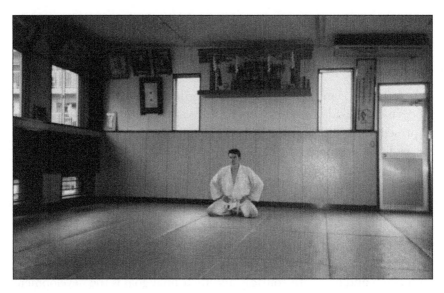

Alone in Kondo Sensei's Shinbukan Dojo in Tokyo. Taking a quiet moment after Sunday training.

showing the distinguished Takeda Clan family emblem, indicating to all who entered that this was a very serious place, and was definitely no sports or social club.

As you entered the building you were met by a simple Zen garden – water dripping from hollow bamboo into a still pond like a steady heartbeat, indicating life and movement. As you went up the stairs, from floor to floor the images and sounds of modern Japan began to change subtly.

The clean and sterile walls of ferro concrete moulded into acute angles of age-old rosewood timber, and the glaring neon and sounds of pachinko dulled to a low hum and were met by the sounds of kiai and the thuds of bodies break falling. As you entered the dojo and stepped onto the hard tatami mats, your stomach would let out a twinge of nervousness. Or was it fear? It may have been both.

The teachings were still true to the founder, Sokaku Takeda – uncompromised, efficient, deadly, and not to be used without responsibility. The Daito Ryu was an elite school worthy of its fame. Back then there was no mass production of black belts, and the dedicated student received intimate instruction from the master and his top students.

For the foreign student, the doors were wide open. Kondo Sensei has been accepting non-Japanese students since 1988. Although Kondo Sensei said that at first he was against taking foreign students, he has so far been impressed with the dedication of the initial overseas students at his dojo.

He feels that if someone really wants to learn Daito Ryu he will teach to the best of his ability, in the hope that the true essence of the art will continue for many years.

But the dedication does not start and end on the dojo floor, for to be able to master the many techniques you have to first master the basics of the Japanese language as no English is spoken.

Kondo Sensei himself has made a lifelong study of the Japanese martial arts. Now in his seventies, he has been studying Daito Ryu for more than 55 years. His first teacher was Hosono Sensei, one of the advanced students of Sokaku Takeda Sensei. After Hosono Sensei passed away, Kondo Sensei trained briefly under Yoshida Sensei, also a senior student of Sokaku Takeda, and finally with the headmaster, the founder's son Tokimune Takeda.

Kondo Sensei is now the only living Daito Ryu Master to hold the Menkyo Kaiden, a license indicating that all knowledge has been transmitted to the receiver, and the Kyoju Dairi, an instructor's certification in the art.

Kondo Sensei has been taught in a direct line from the founder Sokaku Takeda. He feels a responsibility to teach Daito Ryu as taught by the founder, retaining its true value and authenticity. Otherwise the teachings of the Takeda family will fade forever into antiquity. Kondo Sensei is an ardent admirer of the great swordsman and calligrapher Teshuu Sensei, and like Teshuu Sensei believes in the concept of *Shugyo* – periods of intense training to strengthen the body and spirit.

Sensei's strict discipline and etiquette in the dojo, coupled with his uncompromised approach to teaching the techniques of the founder, earned him the nickname Devil Kondo by some of his peers. But make no mistake about it. Back in the late 80s and early 90s, being a student at Kondo Sensei's Shinbukan dojo left you with an incredible feeling that you were experiencing something real and tangible, a real piece of Japanese culture and martial arts history. Not just a hotchpotch of judo and karate techniques stolen from legitimate schools and called ju jitsu, which seemed to be the trend of many Western-based ju jitsu schools.

After spending a couple of months training in Japan in 1989 and 1990, in 1991 I was ready to go in deep. So I made up my mind and left Australia and went to live in Japan to train with the Daito Ryu Aiki ju jitsu full time. I was 28 years old, and very keen to go through total immersion in the hope of finding a new depth of martial arts that I was yet to experience.

Living in Japan on a working visa was the complete experience. After a couple of weeks I had secured a job teaching English, and was confident I would find suitable accommodation. I immediately commenced my training at the Daito Ryu dojo.

Training in Japan was more intensely painful and difficult than any competition I had experienced so far. It was not easy. This was a real dojo, real martial arts. It challenged me physically, mentally and emotionally. The training mats were rock hard, and training was severe. Each move when executed correctly was intensively painful. I faced fear of injury every time I attended.

From the moment I set foot into the dojo, the challenge began. I was thrust head-on into a deep, traditional culture, and to learn the essence of this art I had to become as Japanese as possible. The teachers and students were polite and cordial, and always willing to assist. But I really don't think they expected me to stay.

In fact, I think they were all amazed I had found the dojo in the first place, let alone entered. I was the only foreigner, or at least that's what I thought. For months I was not spoken to, and only took direction by a series of grunts. In the dojo all tuition was in Japanese, and one Japanese student was particularly more abrupt than the others.

After every session, the dojo was cleaned by the students. The most junior (which at that time was me) cleans the toilets. Sumi sempai (sempai is a polite way to address students who are senior to you) took the most pleasure in barking at me in Japanese because the toilets were not good enough. It was hard for me, but I had done worse. It was not going to break me. No

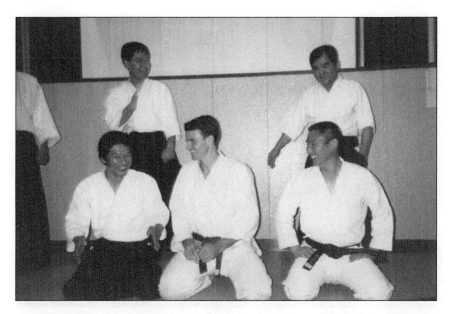

Sharing a light moment after training with Daito Ryu senior students. I love this photo.

way. I started my working career cleaning toilets and digging trenches. I dug deep and constantly reminded myself of the reasons I was there.

Sensei would come to the dojo, and you could feel the tension in the air. I have never met another instructor who had so much power. I felt his power often. For the first three months at the dojo, most of my training was break falling. Break falling is a method of falling when you are thrown by a partner that enables one to land safely. I did hundreds and hundreds of break falls. They threw everything at me and I just kept getting up.

I would get thrown, and instead of thudding me down into the mat they would throw me so I slid across the mat, removing large amounts of skin before I came to a stop. *What was this game? Why were they trying so hard to break me? What was it about me that they did not like? Was it about me? What were they trying to prove?*

My own need to be recognised. My idea that I was already a black belt in other martial arts, and deserved more respect. The need to want to learn quickly, to tick the box. It was all about me. Before they could teach me, they needed to remove my ego, empty my cup. They needed to break me down.

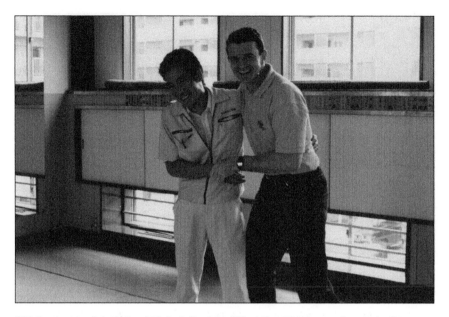

With my mate Mark Sumi. Mark lived in Tokyo for 10 years and was the first non-Japanese to be graded to 3rd Dan Black Belt in Daito Ryu.

After about six weeks everything hurt. I was training most days, and I needed to get over this initial hump. I wanted so badly to quit. My ego was screaming out at me, *Go back home and compete. It's so much easier!* But the longer I was there, the deeper my connection became.

It was Monday, and we had just finished cleaning the dojo. I was rinsing out the clothes when Sumi Sempai came in for his inspection. 'What's up man?' he said in perfect English. I was floored. This was the first time he had spoken to me. I had navigated the past six weeks totally in Japanese.

Mark Sumi was an American-born Japanese raised in California. I had no idea he was American, let alone could speak English. 'Why should you get any special treatment?' he said. 'I had to go through what you did, and it only made me stronger.'

He said, 'You have to learn the language to learn the deeper meaning of the techniques. And in fact, I figured you would have left months ago. It's just too tough for the average person. Man, why are you still here? You have been through hell, man. I had to talk to you. You have paid your dues. It won't be long and Sensei will start talking to you'.

I once heard that the general rule is ju jitsu masters peak in their late 40s or early 50s. I first met Kondo Sensei when he was 49, and looking back I enjoyed my first year of Daito Ryu training with Sensei at his vicious best. My first real introduction to the violent brilliance of Daito Ryu came one Sunday morning three months into my stay.

On the Friday night before, Sensei was leaving the dojo after training when he turned to me and for the first time spoke directly to me. 'Can you come to the dojo for special training this Sunday?' he asked. Naturally, without even thinking I agreed, though I was unsure of the meaning of 'special training'.

That Sunday I realised why I had spent so much time learning how to break fall. It was so I could take Sensei's throws.

Before being thrown by Sensei, he needed to be pretty sure I knew the correct way to land, otherwise I was in a lot of trouble. One Sunday months later, Sensei pulled a throw short, pinning my arms and not allowing me to break fall. I landed full force on my shoulder and neck, and was out for weeks.

On this Sunday, I was introduced to a depth of martial arts that has stayed with me to this day. The power of the lessons, which was not obvious to me then, continues to shape my life now.

When I entered the dojo for the first time I thought I was a pretty good martial artist. At 28 and already a black belt in two other martial arts, I was brash and impatient. I was used to being on the top of the pile and was proud of the way I easily learned new information. I expected to be recognised, and so joining as a white belt and having to start from the beginning again struck a nerve.

On that day, Sensei unleashed his power on me. He asked me to do any attack I wanted. I knew that I was tall and strong, and it was a great chance to prove to Sensei how good I was. I launched my kicks and punches as hard as I could, only to find myself brutally exposed to Sensei's swift counter movements, finding myself time and time again pinned in painful positions or flying through the air.

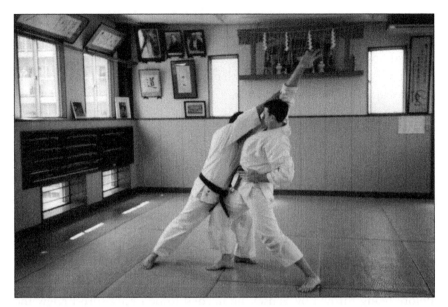

Receiving private lessons from Kondo Sensei.

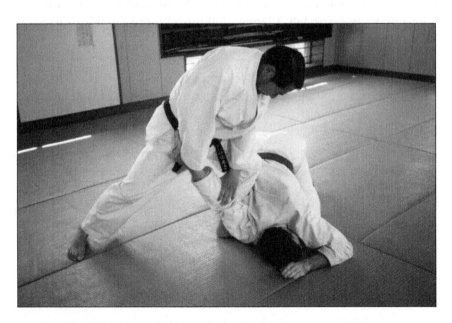

I was blessed to train personally with Kondo Sensei and feel the power of his techniques.

I bled and I cried as Sensei kept repeating, 'Again, again, again'. Each time I landed it became harder and harder for me to stand up. Sensei waited patiently for me, gently adjusting and straightening the framed photos on the wall. There was no malice or brutality. I know this sounds strange, but I felt loved. I finally understood. Initially, Sensei's actions may not always be understood. But a great sensei always has the best intentions for his students.

Sensei needed to break me down and rebuild me from scratch. I could still retain all that I had learned so far, but my blueprint needed to be changed and rebuilt so I could embrace his teachings without the strong attachment to what I had already achieved in the martial arts.

This was a turning point for me, and allowed me to release completely into indulging the experience of living in Japan 100%. I knew then that my obstacle to learning was my resistance to learning a new way of approaching my martial arts. I had been too full of myself to allow any new information in. Sensei knew this, and I finally got what he was doing.

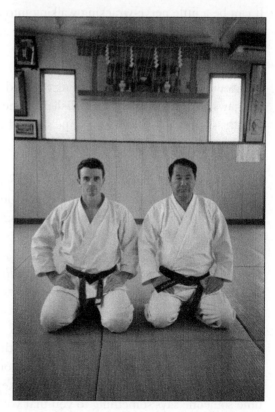

With Kondo Sensei

Submission Arts Wrestling (SAW)

While I was living in Japan in 1991, as well as training in the traditional system of martial arts I also had an interest in the more modern approach to Japanese ju jitsu, which included a freer flowing style and sparring. I was looking through the martial arts magazines in a Tokyo 7-11 when I noticed a small paperback book tucked away in the corner of the racks.

I did not find it. It found me. This has always been the way I have found martial arts schools that would go on to have a significant impact on my life in the most unassuming way.

Usually when I am not researching, I find my best leads in magazines, videos, or in bookshops. The school was Submission Arts Wrestling, and the founder was Hideyuki Aso Sensei. And there was a contact phone number, which I called without hesitation. I first entered SAW in 1991 while I was living in Japan.

It can be a little nerve-wracking walking into a Japanese dojo for the first time, especially into a place so far off the beaten track that the locals themselves have trouble finding the place.

As I walked into the dojo everything stopped. Everyone turned to look at me, jaws slightly dropping in disbelief. Some raised the corners of their mouths slightly in a sneer, and some seemed to be watering at the mouth in expectation of a delicious meal.

All of them had the same look of *My God. A foreigner. Are you insane?* Sometimes when walking into a dojo full of locals I really can understand the feeling of being the lamb before the slaughter.

> *You cannot afford to enter a serious dojo full of young keen fighters too eager to prove your worth, though it does pay to be quietly confident and not show any signs of fear or apprehension. It pays not to overestimate even the white belts, as quite often they are black belts cross-training in a different style.*

In Japanese, there is one word that is worth knowing: *Onegaishimasu*. In its simplest form it means, 'If you please' or 'You would grant me this favour?' It pays to blurt it out to break any tense situations. In fact, every time someone says something to you that you don't understand, a simple

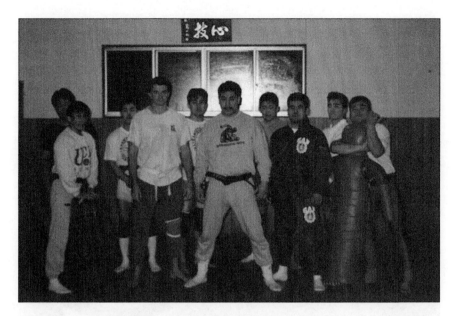

With Aso Sensei, front centre and his students after training. Note that I am wearing a red knee supporter from having my knee injured the night before.

bow of the head and an 'Onegaishimasu' ensures at least you are willing to try.

Of course, it goes without saying that when on the mat, free sparring, doing ground work or whatever, there is no more mister nice guy. Give it your best shot, as this is the only real way to get the respect of your fellow students.

Cross-training in different martial arts has always been popular in Japan. Even if you were totally committed to your current style, you generally had an appreciation and interest in what else was around. Even the most distinguished instructors have Dan grades in several other styles, although these days newer and ever more eclectic styles continue to sprout and take root among the younger generation. It is possible to learn a broad range of skills in different fighting styles under the one school. An instructor with various grades and experience feels the limitations of his traditional training and breaks new ground by setting up his own school.

Submission Arts Wrestling (SAW) is one such school that has broken the mould of the traditional system. An art with a solid foundation in Kodokan judo, wrestling, Sambo wrestling and sumo.

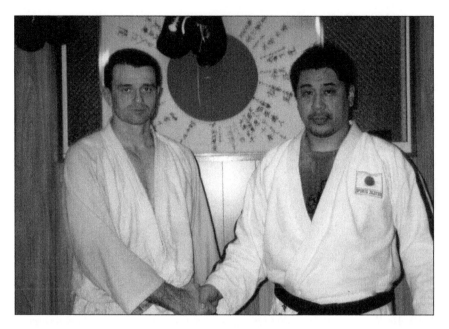

With Aso Sensei. A friendship that has lasted for more than 25 years.

SAW is rapidly growing in popularity in Japan. Many seasoned fighters from all forms of martial arts are attracted to this realistic and progressive form of unrestricted grappling. SAW founder Aso Sensei says, 'Reality is the key, not just in training but also in competition'. Although Aso Sensei agrees that Japan really doesn't have the violence problems of other countries, he is mindful of the modern trend of martial arts toward sports and business, and the eventual extinction of realistic fighting systems altogether.

At the time I met Aso Sensei he was 43 and a solid 100kg, Aso Sensei has a long and experienced background in many forms of fighting. A 5th Dan in Kodokan judo, ex-member of the Japanese national wrestling team and All Japan Masters Wrestling Champion, he has travelled worldwide as player/coach with the Japanese Sambo wrestling team and has many years' experience in karate.

Although Aso Sensei readily admits he cannot explain exactly what *Budo* means (the loose word used to explain Japanese martial arts), he admits it is closely connected to Bushido, or way of the warrior or samurai. He questions this so-called Budo/Bushido spirit and its place in modern

Japanese society, as the samurai era in Japan has long passed. He says Budo is a feeling, a very individual feeling, and according to your training and experience it can be interpreted in many ways.

Aso Sensei sees SAW as a vehicle for learning manners in society, and respect for other people. He stresses that as a student gets stronger, he must control his power. Only the weak readily exploit their skills at a whim. This attitude is reflected in the attitude of his students, who are generally courteous and helpful. (Off the mat, that is. On the mat it's a different story.) Sensei stresses reality and fighting spirit, and the dedication of the students is reflected in their reluctance to submit, even at the risk of a broken arm or a choke out.

An 'Open Submission' competition is held in Tokyo once a year, attracting competitors from all over Japan from every style of grappling. The event is usually dominated by the SAW fighters.

Competition is by no means a focus of training. But if SAW Black Belts are to get recognition and acceptance as a real and serious form of martial arts, then according to Aso Sensei the school must prove its worth against the more established fighting systems.

Chapter 7
Manly Beach, 1992

Arriving home after 12 months of intensive training in Japan was quite a culture shock. After the experience with Kondo Sensei at the three-month mark, I was able to let go of my life in Australia. Other than contact with close family, I closed the door and cut all ties. I was living in Tokyo and began to love it. Other than a couple of other foreign students who were also in the dojo, I avoided contact with all Aussie expats. To get the most out of this experience I wanted to immerse myself fully and learn as much about the martial arts, the language and the culture as I could.

I started to appreciate the beauty in the crowds. No pushing or complaining, just an unwritten acceptance that this is how life works in Japan. Although you were living in a jungle of steel and concrete, you could turn a corner and enter a huge park where the beauty of the spring cherry blossoms live their short but memorable lives, falling from the branch one at a time like a breath out, reminding us that we are all a part of the ever-moving, ever-changing forces of nature.

My body and mind had changed in Japan, honed by hundreds of hours of strict and disciplined training. I felt I belonged in Japan, and was ready to live my life there. But first I needed to go back to Australia to see how I felt after a long time away.

The moment the plane touched down in Sydney I was taken aback by the expanse of the blue sky. It was magnificent. Tokyo is so crowded that you only get snippets of the sky through the buildings masked by the haze. And the spaces between people. In Sydney I could walk freely instead of in a mass throng of controlled movement that left me dizzy. It was the middle of summer 1992, and it was not long before I was riding the waves at Manly beach. As the hard skin and callouses on the joints from the training healed, I quickly slipped back into the laidback Australian lifestyle.

I decided that I would rejoin Qantas as a flight attendant, and continue to work and travel to Japan to continue my training. I also made the decision pretty quickly that I would open up another school and start to teach a style of martial arts that was more in line with what I had been learning over the past couple of years. Once removed from the protective bubble of the all-consuming Japanese experience, I started to enjoy my own training again, only this time I added a few more dimensions.

New martial art, 1992

This new school was the beginning of what would eventually go on to become my life's work, the system I now teach in Sydney: Northstar Ju Jitsu. But at that stage of my life and development, I did not have a clear vision of what my own system would look like. So I simply called the style 'Shinbudo', which could translate to mean 'new martial art'. This was generic enough, and did not pigeonhole me to have to teach a particular style.

I started one afternoon a week in the back meeting room, which was originally the wrestling room at the local community centre run by the police at North Sydney.

Setting up my own martial arts system had its challenges, and it certainly attracted a lot of attention.

Word quickly got around that there was a new and interesting way to learn martial arts. I made many new friends, and met many great like-minded martial artists. But there was also a negative. I had to make sure I was at the top of my game, as I was constantly having to prove the system was effective and worthy to take its place as a new and modern martial art.

Challenges would float in weekly, and if you were training with me back then you would know it was common for me to stop the class and accept the challenge. There were many times when I also accepted challenges outside of the dojo that most people did not know about. It was a great time to be training – exciting, but very scary. The techniques of Shinbudo proved itself against many Australian and world martial arts champions, and was also taken to the edge by many unknowns who had skills and incredible heart.

There are no secrets or shortcuts in martial arts. The only way to get good is through dedication and hard work. That is also the same in life.

Junior

One evening I received a phone call from another martial arts instructor to let me know there was a member of one of Sydney's bikie gangs going around and testing himself against many of the local martial arts schools.

By the time I received the phone call this bikie had managed to impress many of the local martial arts teachers, and was looking for his next challenge. This martial arts instructor who called me had just been visited by the bikie, and managed to talk his way out of a confrontation by kindly giving my details. So he was calling me to warn me.

Sure enough, the following Saturday we had just commenced training when this man mountain appeared at the dojo door in full bikie colours. He stood there and demanded to see Andrew Dickinson. He looked me squarely in the eye and said, 'Are you fighting today?'

'I am now,' I said.

As he walked into the dojo, I discreetly locked the door behind him, ensuring that only the winner would walk out.

This was often the one thing that separated me from the various challengers. I was always deadly serious and willing to put it all on the line.

'Junior' was the sergeant-at-arms for one of the larger bike clubs at the time. He was a massive lump of muscle, well over 190cm and weighing in at over 120kg. He had a red goatee beard and a plait of red hair that extended to his waist. He had a fierce reputation and was well respected by other bikie gangs, not to mention he had already mixed it with several other top martial arts instructors.

Seeing him standing there, of course I was scared. I could feel the mix of fear and adrenalin surge through my body. On the outside I was calm and relaxed, but on the inside I was screaming and wanted to run in the opposite direction as fast as possible.

> *Fear is the protector. It is the natural defence mechanism set off by the body in order to survive. To not feel any fear when faced with danger is more of a worry. Fear is never the problem. It is how you react to the fear. Some people let it cripple them, others can still functional efficiently.*

I simply said, 'You are welcome to join us', to which he took off his jacket, shoes and socks and walked onto the mat wearing jeans and a t-shirt. As it was our regular sparring session, there was a range of belts. Junior joined the end of the line and made short work of several brown belts, literally picking them up and slamming them into the mats. I knew I had to put a stop to this, and I had to do it fast.

We stood in front of each other, and I could feel his fear. I knew he was unpredictably dangerous, and that this would be a dirty scrap if I let it go on.

I bowed. He stood and glared. As he took one step towards me I launched a front leg turning kick that landed square on his jaw. The sound of my foot smashing into his face stopped the entire room. His eyes dimmed as he dropped to both knees. I quickly followed up by rushing him onto the ground and drawing his long plait around his neck continued to choke him with his own hair. I clearly remember him trying to find my eyes with his thumbs as he slowly became limp.

When I finally let go of him, he was sound asleep. A minute or so later, as he was trying to crawl on all fours back to the door, my younger brother (also a black belt) said, 'Oh no you don't. We have not finished with you yet'.

Junior took a terrible pounding that day. He was very quiet by the end of it, and politely excused himself as we unlocked the door and let him out.

The following Monday he was back at the dojo. I thought, *Here we go again.* But to my surprise he was dressed in normal gear and looked completely different from the first time I met him. He extended his hand and requested to become my student.

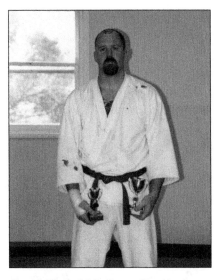

Junior had been looking for a teacher who could tame him, and he found that in our school. He was humble and respectful, so I allowed

David 'Junior' Newham after winning an interclub competition.

him to join as a white belt. Junior trained with us for five years, almost gaining a black belt. Though our worlds were different, we respected each other. I did not really understand what it meant to be a Hells Angel, and the only condition was that he leave that world behind when he came to train. I also made it very clear that he was not allowed to use any martial arts that I taught him in any fights with other bikies or anyone else outside of the dojo, which did become quite difficult to control.

Junior became my close friend. He was respected and loved by many in the dojo. Years later, Junior and I would often laugh as we would relive the first time we met. He would say he knew that he was in trouble the moment he laid eyes on me, which was funny as I thought the same thing. He never saw the kick, so he never knew what hit him. All he would say is that he had never been hit so hard.

One winter morning in 1998, as I was arriving back from Japan, I got the terrible news that Junior had been murdered. It was a huge blow to all who knew him. A seemingly unprovoked attack by a gunman who was intent on killing him. Junior kept us all well protected from his other world, so I never knew the depth of his darker side, though I had a healthy respect for his love of his bikie life. I loved him like a brother, and accepted him for his humanness.

Learn one system, then learn the counters to the same system. Learn the moves of the boxer, then learn how to nullify the boxer by learning a new system. Turn the system back on itself and expose its weakness.

Training evolution

Over my many years of martial arts training, I became an excellent kicker – strong, fast and precise. But there were plenty of fighters who were better. So if I sensed I was losing against a superior kicker, I needed to develop an immediate change in fighting strategy that would cut the kicker to pieces.

I turned my technique against itself and looked for flaws and weaknesses within my kicking game. The main influence in the development of learning how to defend against kicks was Aso Sensei and his Submission Arts Wrestling (SAW).

The first chance I got to test my theory was against four-time world kickboxing champion and Commonwealth boxing champion Adam Watt. I had known Adam for years, and we were good mates. He was training for the World Thai Boxing title against Dutch great Rob Kaman, and asked if he could meet and spar with me for preparation. I agreed. So every morning we would meet at the North Sydney PCYC in what was the original downstairs dojo and do at least six rounds of sparring.

To tell you the truth, I was completely outclassed in all areas of kicking, punching and general fitness. Adam was at the height of his game, and to be fair I had to play his game. My sparring had developed into a complete system of fighting that could mould itself based on the weakness of my opponent. So after a couple of days of having the stuffing knocked out of me I asked Adam if we could do some no-rules fighting. Within a blink I caught Adam's long powerful turning kick and slammed him down onto his back, quickly mounted to ground position three and applied a submission. Just to show it was no fluke, I did it again.

The next round Adam peppered me with fast head punches that I could not avoid. So to his delight I rushed in, only to be welcomed by a vice-like neck clinch and a barrage of knees I could not escape.

Round four I had a plan. I knew I could not escape his devastating knee assault, so I decided to embrace it. Adam had learned to keep his kicks down, but I was waiting for the knees. It did not take Adam long to cover the distance between us, but this time I welcomed him. He clinched both his arms around my neck and proceeded to go to work with the knees.

The first one I managed to block. The second one caught me right in the solar plexus, knocking the wind out of me. But I managed to grab his thigh above the knee. I wrapped both my arms around his knee, and while he was hopping on one leg and hitting me at the same time in the back of the head, I waited and got my breath back, which took about three seconds. Then with one explosive action I palmed Adam's leg so that instead of me being front-on to Adam I was now side-on, at the same time sweeping his standing leg out from under him. I quickly took control on the ground.

I appreciated that Adam allowed me to try some different types of sparring, and it was indicative of the great champion that he was.

Time to compete again, 1992

Since returning from living in Japan, I began to feel more and more that there was unfinished business in the competitive ring. I had fantasies about competing in the tough Daido Juku Karate Championships in Japan. But the full-head contact, and wearing the plastic head protector that was shaped like a bubble, just was not my thing.

It was 1992, and it was the very beginning of the concept of training in several martial arts and combining their best techniques into a more complete style of fighting. Japan had been hosting the concept of limited-rules fighting for many years, but the rest of the world was slow to embrace the idea. My first try was at a Submission Arts Wrestling competition in Nagoya Japan in 1992.

It was great working as a flight attendant again, particularly after living in Japan. I was able to travel to and from Japan and continue my training there. It just so happened that the Nagoya competition was on at the same time as a 24-hour layover I had with work, so I decided to go for it.

It was risky business, as I knew injuries were common in the Submission Arts Wrestling competitions. And I did not exactly have the blessing of the airline I was working for.

I was quite nervous, as this was the first time I had competed in Japan and my first time competing in a No-Gi (shorts and t-shirt instead of the standard martial arts uniform) submission competition. There were fighters from all over Japan representing many different forms of grappling including judo, Sambo and BJJ, as well as many freestyle systems that were combinations of several grappling systems.

And then there was me, the only non-Japanese fighter there.

I was made to feel welcome, and already knew several of the fighters from the training I had experienced previously in Japan. The fights started in a frenzy of legs, arms and bodies. Already knees were popped and shoulders were torn. Watching this was no easy feat as I had to stay injury-free so I could work home that night.

Though I had made a strong resolve to compete again, it took all my strength to stay committed to this path. I had registered and lost my nerve a couple of times, but this time I was determined. Just turning up, registering and weighing in for the competition, I felt a great sense of accomplishment. And no matter what the outcome, I felt I had overcome a huge barrier.

My first fight was against a freestyle grappler. It felt quite strange fighting without any kicks or punches, so I was quite out of my comfort zone. The fight quickly fell to the ground where I was able to take control. Though I was ahead on points, I finished my opponent off with a painful arm lock, winning the fight.

My next fight was against Kawamura-san, a tough, skilled martial artist. Kawamura-san hooked my front leg and swept it out from under me. I felt the crack in my ankle as my body hit the mat. I was in fight mode, so I ignored the pain and in the back of my mind I just hoped it was not bad. I hobbled to the end of the bout and lost by a respectful two points. Kawamura-san went on to win the Middleweight All Japan Ju Jitsu Championship, and a silver in the 1996 World Sports Ju Jitsu Championships in Canada.

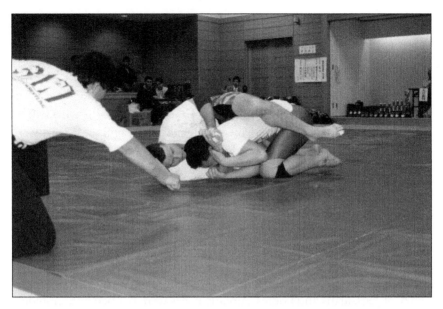

Fighting Kawamura-san in the SAW Championships in Nagoya Japan.

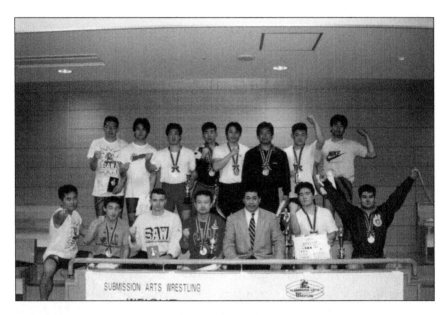

Sitting with Aso Sensei and the winners in Nagoya Japan.

The competition finished on schedule, so I had enough time to ice my swollen ankle in my hotel room before my night shift home. The good news was I could stand up. The bad news was it was painful to walk. My buddy carried my bag for me, and I limped onto the aircraft. There was no way I could work. Lucky for me the crew were kind as they were told I had just twisted my ankle jogging. They packed ice onto my foot, threw a blanket over me and I slept all the way home.

That was not the first and only time I competed when on duty as a flight attendant. In fact, it was not so much the competing that was the problem but the injuries in training when overseas. Like the time I had my front teeth elbowed out in Los Angeles.

I was training regularly with the Machado Brothers BJJ school in Redondo, and on this one occasion I was wrestling with another white belt who was very strong and aggressive. His movement was wild and unpredictable. I used to enjoy training with raw but strong beginners as they don't follow predictable patterns of trained students, and quite often they can catch you with something totally random.

This was a great way to prepare for a street fight. At my own classes, I used to love the challenge of a big strong beginner, especially rugby players. I would always make a point to spar with them during the class.

Back to the Machado class. My opponent spun quickly and caught me with a short hard elbow to the mouth, knocking out my front teeth. This was not a good look, and working home from LA as a flight attendant would be near impossible.

Rigan Machado had a great idea. One of his students owned a cosmetic dentistry clinic close by. The problem was it was already 8pm. Rigan's magic in organising the dentist was impressive. It was almost as good as his ju jitsu. An hour later we were at the dental clinic having the roots removed and the teeth glued back into position. They would at least survive the trip back to Australia.

I had problems with my front teeth for many years. If only I had worn a mouth guard.

Taking SAW a step further

The SAW Special Rule competition in Tokyo was a great way for me to test my skills in a format that combined the throws and ground fighting of wrestling and judo with the kicking and punching skills of taekwondo and kickboxing. This was a No-Gi, bare knuckle event in a boxing ring, and was televised on Tokyo Television. The fight was two five-minute rounds, which would be a new experience for me as the longest I had experienced in previous competitions was three three-minute rounds.

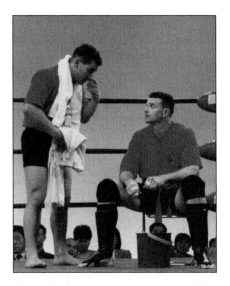

Calm in between rounds with Dimi Tops.

To win I knew I had to get a submission or knock my opponent out. You see, to win in Japan you really have to be on your game. Back when I had this fight I had been training for some years with the Japanese, so they were used to me and I had proven myself in their dojo. This style of fighting was quite new, and I was very excited to be able to try my all-round fighting style in Japan.

I was very nervous, but had trained hard. Tachi san, my opponent, was very experienced and seemed to have no fear. During the first round Tachi kicked my legs hard. That got my attention. I scored well, mixing up my kicks with throwing techniques, and was feeling relaxed and comfortable at the end of the first round.

In the second round I changed my stance slightly so I could block his leg kicks. The moment Tachi saw me switch stance he delivered a knee to my head that rocked me. I did not go down, but because I was seeing double I kept my distance in order to recover. This would have been a great opportunity for Tachi to knock me out as I was really struggling.

I quickly recovered and knew I had to finish him. The first chance I got I took him down to the ground, got into a good position, and locked his arm up in a submission move on his elbow. I was slowly stretching his elbow, and I could feel the sinews in his joint start to snap. I was not prepared to break his arm, and was just about to let him go when he submitted by tapping the rope of the ring.

Feeling a wave of exhilaration mixed with relief, I stood up and was awarded the fight. As I was about to climb out of the ring and make my out, the centre referee got a message on his headset from the officials that we were to continue fighting. Keeping a cool head was all part of the training, so I did not complain and just got on with it.

I was well ahead on points, but as I had just experienced that was no guarantee of a win. I had to finish strong. The final bell rang with me straddled on top of Tachi, sliding my elbows across his face. It took a while for Tachi to regain his feet, and when he did he was bloodied and bruised. With points 10-0 in my favour they awarded me the win. It was a great all-round experience, and I was very happy to eventually win. Competing in Japan, you never know what is coming your way. But that is part of the challenge.

Within the softness of Japanese ju jitsu there is great strength in yielding, flowing, redirecting. Approaching conflict with an attitude of forgiveness instead of aggression. Like water, like the willow. You don't have to forgive the act, but you can forgive the person.

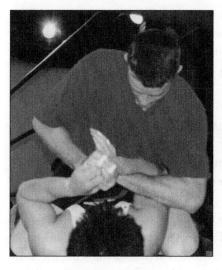 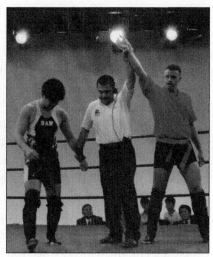

On top of Tachi san, looking for an arm lock to finish the fight.

Taking the points decision. 10-0.

Black belt surprise

One of my most memorable gradings was for my 1st Dan black belt in Daito Ryu Aiki ju jitsu in July 1996. And it was a grading that caught me completely by surprise.

Though not living in Japan at the time, I had spent quite a lot of time up there, often going up every other weekend and training then coming back to Sydney.

I had spent the 12 months living and training in Japan in 1991, and by the end of the 12 months was awarded a brown belt 3rd kyu in Daito Ryu Aiki ju jitsu. So there were two more grades I would need to pass before I was eligible to try for the black belt. As there was no Daito Ryu under Kondo Sensei anywhere but in Tokyo, it meant I had to travel backward and forwards during work with the airline, my downtime from work and on my holidays.

It took me four years, but I completed the next two grades and was finally able to sit for my black belt test. I would just have to wait for Kondo Sensei to approve my application. This was very important to me, as I would be the first Australian to be awarded a Daito Ryu Aiki Ju Jitsu black belt under Kondo Sensei.

This time I was on one of my regular scheduled training visits, but was nowhere near ready to take the tough black belt grading. In fact, it was a grading I was dreading, and wanted to put it off for as long as possible. Daito Ryu is a very hard and disciplined form of martial arts, and up until the time I did my grading there was only one other non-Japanese student graded to black belt before me: Mark Sumi.

Sydney to Tokyo is about nine hours through the night, and I left a Sydney winter to arrive at the onslaught of a very hot and humid Japanese summer. Training was scheduled for 10am, so I quickly caught the train from Narita airport. Getting the train at Narita is always a bonus, as it is the first station on the line and you get the pick of the best seats.

The trains quickly fill up. In fact, fill up is an understatement. They get so full that you can feel the air being pushed out of your body as more and more people are crammed in. So while you have the best pick on the seats, the most important thing is to know what side of the train you are going to get off on, particularly if you have bags, and to position yourself close to the door.

The key to getting off the crowded train is to stand and start gently pushing. It's okay to push, as long as it is not done in an aggressive manner. Gently push. If you are not getting anywhere, push a little harder until people start to move out of your way. You have to stay calm and keep a smile on your face. People will generally spill out onto the platform to make way for you. No-one is offended by this. It's just what is needed to get off the train.

After spilling onto the platform at Shinkoiwa station there was a stillness as the train so full of life disappeared. I almost felt stranded, left behind alone on the empty platform, sweat massing under my winter clothes in the bite of Tokyo summer. The desire to just sit and wait for the next train home immediately crossed my mind. It always does when I first arrive at Shinkoiwa. It's just my old friend fear trying to protect me from the mental and physical pain Daito Ryu brings.

The body just seems to drive itself. There is no more thinking about should I or shouldn't I? The legs walk, the body moves, and then the mind follows. Funny, it should be the other way around – the mind deciding the action of the body. This was one of my first very small insights into the mind not being the one in control.

Deep within, a decision had been made. And no amount of thinking was going to change the outcome. Once a course of action has been decided by something deeper than just everyday thinking it becomes a soul choice, and needs to be followed through on completely, sometimes against all logic.

I don't know why I am doing this. But there is something deeper within that understands I just have to go through with it. From this deeper drive within the outcome, be it positive or negative, comes a profound learning that enhances the spirit, and prepares you for more.

The effort to get to the dojo is a test in itself, so arriving I always feel a sense of achievement. This is not something I love and can't wait to do. It's hard to explain. On this day I met up with my good friend and great exponent of ju jitsu Phil Hinshelwood, who just happened to be in Tokyo at the same time. I invited him to tag along to the dojo to watch the training session.

We arrived at the dojo after a brisk 20-minute walk from the station. My friend and Daito Ryu black belt Mark Sumi was there to meet me as usual. It appeared that this was just going to be a regular training session. Kondo Sensei was all business as Mark and I started to warm up.

Part of the warm up was for Mark to throw me. It is called *ukemi*. You take your partners wrists, and he throws you by flipping you in the air landing hard on the mat. The tatami mats in the dojo were hard and unforgiving. The slightest misthrow from Mark or lack of commitment from me would quickly result in injury. So Mark began by asking me how many times I would like to be thrown, and before I could reply he said 30 times should be enough.

Bearing in mind that I had not slept, and had come straight to the dojo from Australia, I was exhausted after only 10 throws. Mark and I then trained doing the techniques for an hour. I knew the techniques very well, as I did many hours of small group lessons with Sensei every Sunday when I was living in Tokyo.

After about an hour, Amano Sempai arrived in his uniform. I thought this was a little strange, as it was Saturday and Amano usually works on Saturdays. It was great to have him in the dojo as he is such a powerful force and always so happy. Sensei suddenly turned to me and said, 'Andy, you will now do your black belt test'. I was stunned as I really had not been prepared for this. But I knew I had no choice.

We drilled technique after technique, with Mark relentless in his attack. I was struggling to focus but kept on going. At intervals during the techniques Sensei would fire off questions in Japanese asking me to explain in detail the theory behind each move, and my responses all had to be in Japanese. I was on autopilot, just surviving and responding to what was asked of me.

Everyone who grades for black belt in Daito Ryu has to do 100 break falls by being thrown 100 times. So I knew what was coming. I believe this is one of the hardest tests that you can ever do. It was for me, anyway. Every time you stand you are thrown back onto the floor.

It is a real test of courage, resilience and determination. No rest and no stopping, my body screaming out to stop. I was ready to quit after 30

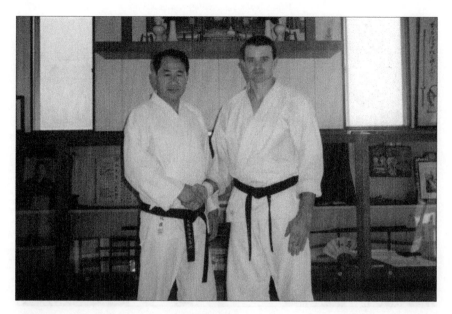

With Kondo Sensei at his dojo in Tokyo Japan.

throws, but something so deep, so primal, moved me from within. I had no control. My mind and body were moving as one. I was simply an observer of the action. The pain in my legs and arms seemed like they belonged to someone else. I was completely lost in the motion.

The longer it went on the more Mark increased the intensity, determined to break me. The count was lost in a blur at eternity. I had no idea what the number was, but then it all stopped. I kept on standing, refusing to stop. I had to make 100. I had to do it. Mark bowed and sat on his knees facing Sensei, indicating that we had finished. I made the 100 without realising it.

I dropped to my knees and bowed deeply to Sensei, then to Mark. The grading was over, and I had passed. It was an honour to be privately graded by Sensei. It was 10 years since I had first stepped into Kondo Sensei's dojo. Ten years of travelling to Japan and back. This was the only way it was ever going to happen, and Sensei knew it.

Accept change. In fighting you have to adapt and move quickly. The instant you get set in your ways, you get hit. This is a great metaphor for living. If you are too set into believing your reality will never change, when it does change there is incredible suffering.

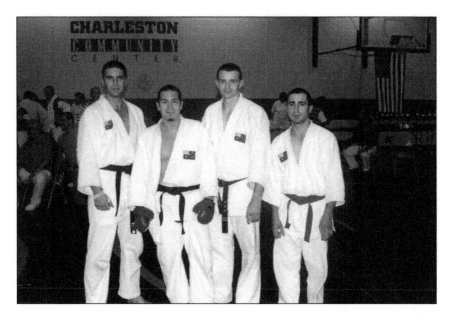

A tough bunch of Aussie mates taking on the best sports ju jitsu fighters. L-R: Carl Safar,
Dimi Tops, me and Peter Barbanera.

West Virginia, 1996

In early 1996 I was elected to be the vice-chairman of the International
Sports Ju Jitsu Association (ISJA) by Sports Ju Jitsu chairman and
MMA pioneer Ernie Boggs. As the first International Sports Ju Jitsu
Championships was in October in West Virginia, I put a team together
of the best fighters who were training with me at the time. A tough bunch
of black belts who were also my mates: Dimi Tops, Carl Safar and Peter
Barbenera. We were just a group of rough Aussie lads about to compete
against the world's best ju jitsu fighters ever assembled.

We arrived at West Virginia after a mammoth flight from Sydney. Suitably
jetlagged, we checked into the motel close to the competition venue. Other
than Carl who was the super heavyweight, the rest of us had to cut weight
to make the weigh-in for the category we were fighting in. It was torture.
To be in the USA and for the first few days only eat salad and sip water.

We all made weight the day before the competition. I was nervous, and spent
the entire night before the competition churning over possible scenarios
and outcomes. It was a complete waste of time, as I have come to learn

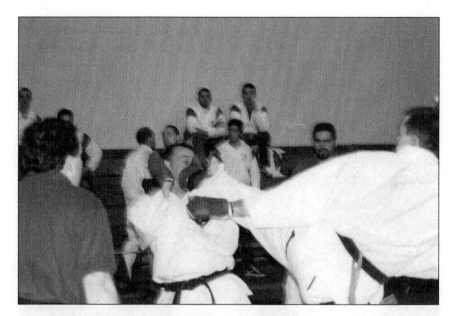

Fighting the tough Argentinian Captain, Claudio Palumbo.

that trying to predict any outcome just wastes precious time in the present moment. We spend so much of our lives planning for the future or mulling over the past that we miss the real essence of life here and now. As it was, if I knew what was in store for me I would have probably run for my life.

I was the first fight of the day. The bout was against the very experienced Argentinian captain Claudia Palumbo. This was to be right up there as one of the toughest fights of my life. Without a doubt, Claudio wanted to kill me. He hit me hard and was relentless, easily winning the first round. I was short of breath and struggling. I think that the jetlag and cutting of weight took its toll as my body was heavy and slow to respond. The second round was just a blur. Not only did I win the round, I had somehow scored enough points to win the fight. But the fight really took it out of me, and I had to regroup quickly to take on Blair Phillips, ex-heavyweight world champion.

At this high level of fighting, there were plenty of injuries. People were dropping all over the place, with two ambulances running a shuttle back and forth to the hospital. The entire team knew the seriousness of what we were doing, and knew the only way to avoid injury was to fight hard. Each of us fighting with all our hearts, maybe not winning but gaining the respect of all we came into contact with.

I put everything into my fight with Blair, losing the first round but winning the second, taking the fight to a draw. We fought two rounds of extra time. I was done, but I fought my heart out. One thing I have learned about myself through hardship is that I have the ability to stand tall and dig deep, *real* deep, when faced with overwhelming odds.

Even though Blair got the final decision, he later told me he thought I had won, and that it was one of his toughest fights.

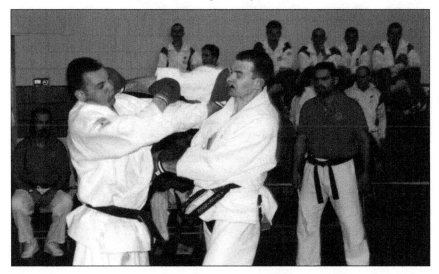

Fighting against Claudio was intense. I felt I was fighting for my life.

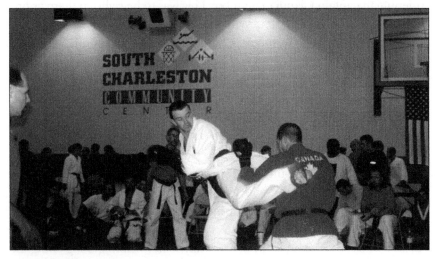

Missing with a kick against Canadian champion Blair Phillips.

My son Tom

Hisako, my first wife, and I always planned on having children. I was sure I was ready, and I figure all new parents say the same. But nothing prepared me for the actuality of parenthood.

During the first months of pregnancy Hisako suffered terrible nausea and was unable to look after herself. At six months, Tom decided he'd had enough of waiting and made signs he was ready to be born. So on the advice of our specialist she needed to remain lying down and looked after. We were living in Australia, but as I was away a lot of the time working for Qantas we decided the best option would be for Hisako to be looked after by her family in Tokyo.

On the morning of the 5th of July 1997 I was heading to Osaka with work, so I called Hisako to see if she was okay. She had been resting in Tokyo at her mother's house for the past few weeks, and I was reassured that all was stable and running to plan. Hisako was at 37 weeks, and was looking forward to a natural birth at 40 weeks.

But Tom had other plans.

I arrived at Osaka International Airport at around 5.30pm after a long day's work. I was looking forward to relaxing in the hotel. I would call Hisako once I arrived and was settled in my room just to check in and see how she was.

As soon as the front door of the Qantas 767 was opened I got a message that Hisako had gone into labour and to come to Tokyo as soon as possible. I immediately called Qantas in Sydney to tell them my son was being born and to ask permission to fly to Tokyo. But I was not prepared for the frosty reception I received. I was basically told I had to stay in Osaka and make sure I was working back as scheduled the following night. If I didn't, I would be stood down.

I ignored all that.

My crew and the Qantas ground staff in Osaka were terrific. We quickly booked a ticket for the hour-long flight to Tokyo, and I was on my way. I just hoped I would make it for the birth.

I arrived at Haneda Airport in Tokyo, and jumped straight into a taxi and headed towards the Red Cross hospital. I had no idea at this stage whether I would be in time for the birth or not. I finally arrived at the hospital at 9.30pm. Tom was born at 3.10am the next morning on the 6th of July 1997, three weeks early. I was blessed that I made the birth.

Straight after the birth the baby is taken by the midwife, washed, wrapped, then given to the father while the obstetrician cleans the mother up. So I was sitting alone with this incredible bundle of new life, tears streaming down my face as I made a promise to my newborn son. I promised that no matter what happened in life, I would always be there for him.

Now committing to your child may sound like a natural thing to do for a parent. But I was making a promise that I would never break. I did not want to repeat the same pattern of my parents and leave Tom with the same insecurities I had as a child.

The birth of Tom, and the experience of being a father, has been and still is the greatest gift. Being a good, committed and loving father has been my greatest accomplishment.

Chapter 8
London, February 1998

F or most of the experiences I had in other countries I was alone. I
generally trained and prepared alone, and relied on my own counsel
to make decisions. I was a pioneer of sorts, and although I got into
some dangerous situations I got a real thrill out of not only surviving but
actually thriving under pressure. I would not go out of my way to place
myself in needless danger. But in many situations, if I was not prepared
and not cautious I could have easily been in trouble.

I was scheduled to work on a flight to London, and it just so happened
that the British Fighting Grand Prix was on. As I was born in England it
was always on my mind that it would be an honour to fight on home soil.
So I contacted my friend Tom Mullins from the English Sports Ju Jitsu
Association to see if it was at all possible.

The Grand Prix was a fight night, with the best fighters in sports ju jitsu from
England, Scotland and Wales matched against each other. I knew many of
the British fighters, and their standard was excellent. Tom Mullins agreed,
and said if I could make it he would be delighted to have me. The pieces
seemed to fall together effortlessly. I had a 36-hour layover in London that
gave me just enough time to compete then work back to Sydney.

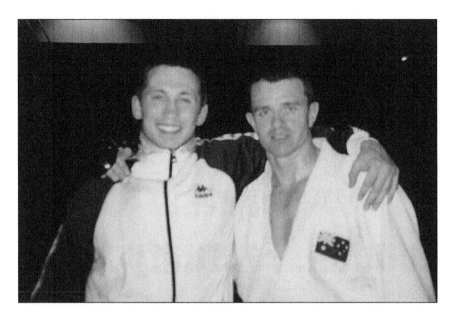

Sports Ju Jitsu Legend Gary Turner sat in my corner while in Yorkshire.

I trained hard for the competition, and was confident I would survive. For the past few years I had been using a method of training that when followed to the letter enabled me to peak exactly on competition day no matter where I was or what time it was. I proved this system worked time and time again, peaking in England, Canada and Japan on minimum sleep without adjusting for time zones, and in completely different seasons.

I arrived in London on the Friday evening after a long flight from Bangkok, ate dinner and then tried to sleep. Like all competitions I have entered, sooner or later fear starts to push its way forward. For me it was always the night before, and I rarely slept before a competition. I still had no idea who I was fighting, and travelling to the other side of the world for a six-minute fight meant losing was not an option.

My friend and World Ju Jitsu Champion Gary Turner picked me up at 9am from the hotel in London for the drive north to Yorkshire. The fights were not due to start until Saturday evening, so it was a very long day and I was tired from lack of sleep.

I was beginning to wonder why I was doing this. But something deep within me always pushed me that last step. The self-doubt, fear, and all the reasons why I should just pack up and catch the first train back to London started to come, wave after wave. The strength of conviction to face my fear dominated any negatives, and I was driven to complete the task regardless of the outcome.

I just had to do it. It is amazing that your experiences and influences during childhood can become such a driving force throughout life.

> *I have come to trust that life is a gift that gives us opportunities to face the challenges that present themselves so we can grow spiritually. Of course, many do not have the desire to face such challenges, or live life unaware that they exist.*

At last the fights started. The bouts were ferocious. I went through my warmup, breathing and remaining calm. Feeling the nerves rising, I knew that if left uncontrolled they would spiral me down and I would start doubting myself. It took all of my inner strength to stay composed, even though there was already a war going on inside my head.

My opponent was a large Yorkshire lad. He kept his distance, but when he moved in he was fast and his punches were scoring. I was getting frustrated. I tried to counter quickly, but my timing was off and he was too fast. He easily won the first round. I sat in my corner at the end of the round and Gary, who was my corner man in no uncertain terms, reminded me that I did not come all this way to lose.

The second round started, and I knew I had to get a quick submission. I feinted a punch with my left, and immediately followed with a high left turning kick that caught him flush on the chin. I shot in and swept him onto the ground, taking side control. His arm came up and I fell onto it applying an arm lock. There was no way I was going to let it go. In pain he quickly submitted by tapping with his free hand. No-one was hurt, and it was a good fight. It was a good win.

We left Yorkshire late that evening and Gary dropped me back to the hotel in London. I managed a couple of hours sleep before getting ready for the long flight home. It had been an experience I would not forget in a hurry. Work to London, 36-hour layover, fight, win, then work home.

All Japan Ju Jitsu Championship, July 1998

At the All Japan Ju Jitsu Championships in 1998 I pushed it to the limit. The competition was in July, so straight off I was going from a freezing cold Australian winter into the middle of a hot and humid Tokyo summer. I arrived from Sydney on the Saturday before the tournament. I knew I was cutting it fine by arriving the day before, but that was how I did things. I was looking forward to the chance to compete in Japan again, and to challenge myself against fighters from all styles from all over the country.

I spent the Saturday morning relaxing at my favourite park, Shinjuku Koen, which was a short stroll from my hotel. It is an amazing place – so still and quiet, except for the haunting squawk of the crows that circle eerily yet elegantly above. The park is a complete contrast from the rest of Tokyo.

I walked back to the hotel through the back streets of Shinjuku, close to my favourite sounding station Takadanababa. I then made my way through Kabookicho, a maze of nightclubs, noisy Pachinko parlours, neon lights and street vendors spruiking their fresh produce. Coming back to Japan after living there in 1991, I always felt quite at home.

Japan is so unique. It has always amazed me how a population of 127 million people can be crammed into a country the size of the east coast of Australia, yet seemingly live in harmony with nature and each other. I was never obsessed by Japan as some people are, losing their own identity and becoming more Japanese than the Japanese themselves. I tended to stay away from the expats living in Japan, preferring the company of my Japanese friends.

On Sunday morning I was up early and ate a light Japanese-style breakfast of rice, salmon and miso soup. Then I made my way to the famous Shinjuku station for the 45-minute ride north of Tokyo to the city of Saitama.

I stepped out of the air-conditioned train and was taken aback by the wall of heat. At least there would be air-conditioning at the competition venue. I arrived at the sports centre, which was only a short stroll from the station, and quickly changed for the weigh-in. The fighters are weighed before the competition to make sure they are competing in the correct weight category. I like the idea of weighing in on the day of competition as it keeps fighters close to their fighting weight. I was competing in the 75-90kg heavyweight class, and I weighed in at 90kg on the dot.

The temperature inside the hall was more than 40 degrees Celsius. And no aircon. I had competed in Thailand under the same conditions years ago, so I was confident I could handle it. Fighters from all styles of martial arts were gathered from all over Japan. I was the only non-Japanese fighter, but I knew some of the competitors and officials having competed and trained in Japan many times.

The tournament was full contact with throws and ground fighting. A tough and robust system of fighting, pitting various styles against each other. The 20 fighters in the heavyweight division were fit, strong and hungry for action. I was quietly confident, as I had put in a solid three months of preparation for this competition and was in great shape.

My first fight was up against a submission fighter affectionately known as Beatle. I had grappled with him once or twice, and although he was heavy and strong I never felt worried, so I was preparing for an easy match.

I should have known better. There is always an X factor when competing, and so-called mediocre fighters can take you by surprise.

Beatle came at me hard, and I responded by going hard back. I could not believe it. I was quickly drained of all energy and strength, probably a combination of the long flight, the heat and nerves. Beatle was short and tough, and if I was not super careful he was going to knock me out.

Damn I hate being in this position. The lone wolf. No coach or training partners, no support from the spectators, just the high-pitched staccato of the Japanese pushing Beatle to finish me off. This just added to the challenge.

It was not that I enjoyed being alone, or that I was at my best being alone. It was more that I knew what I was looking for, and had an unshakable trust in my ability to be able to choose the experiences that aligned with my personal journey. Everyone has their own personal journey. It is just more obvious to some than others. I was driven not just to be the best I could be, but to also understand deep in my heart that I accepted myself for who I was and was respected as a martial artist.

The two-minute round seemed like an eternity. I just made it to my stool and sat alone as I regrouped. *I've trained, I've prepared, and I definitely have not come all this way to lose against Beatle in the first round.*

It takes a champion mindset to reprogram yourself in 30 seconds to win, especially after the punishment I took in round one. I was way behind on points, and the only way I was going to win was by knockout.

This scenario – losing the first round and having to do a Rocky-like comeback to win – seems to have become an unconscious pattern in so many of my fights. So as I sat by myself waiting for the second round to start, I leveraged all of my training to realign the reasons I was there – being the only non-Japanese fighter, and to have the honour of winning such an important event – and what I needed to do to win.

As the second round started, I was up on my toes and feeling great. I felt that the first round had warmed me up, settled the nerves, and given me a large enough scare to now know what to do.

Beatle lunged forward. I slipped to the side and spun, launching a very powerful spinning back kick that caught him squarely in the stomach.

For an instant he just stood still, and I was wondering in that moment if he had felt it at all. A surge of panic raced through my body. If that kick did not hurt him nothing would. He grabbed his stomach and dropped to his knees, groaning. The referee stopped the fight immediately, raising my arm in victory. What a relief.

I floated through my next fights up on my toes and dancing into the final. This really was the fight of my life. I was so excited to be in the final. I watched the other fighter demolish his opponents as he rampaged into the final. He was a university judo champion, and once he got you in his grip it was just a matter of time before he had you in a vulnerable position and tossed you like a rag doll.

Preparing for the final against the judo fighter, I knew that if he got a hold of me he would throw me hard. I had done judo for five years at Sydney University, but I was way out of his league. So I played to my strengths: hitting him hard every time he was in range. He quickly got

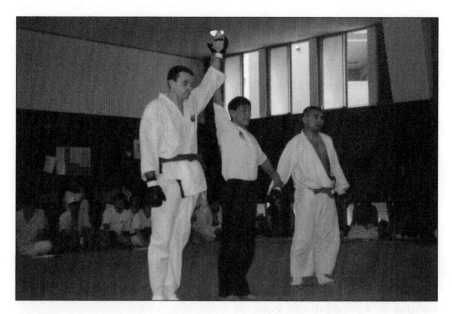

Winning a tough fight against Beatle.

frustrated, losing his nerve and resorting to rushing in, which only made it worse for him.

In the first few seconds of the fight I kicked him hard in the head. It would have knocked over a bull, but he just shrugged it off, spat out his mouth guard and kept walking forward. He was one tough fighter.

The key to winning this fight was being in great shape so I was constantly on the move, and using kicks and punches from every angle. Sometimes, or should I say rarely, all the parts of a fight just fall into place. The fitness, the technique, the mindset and not being crippled by fear all align. This was by far the best I have fought in any competition.

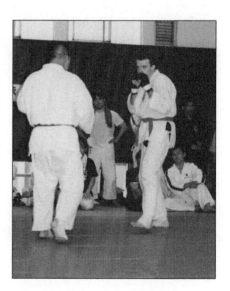

The final fight of the All Japan Ju Jitsu Championships.

I was 35, and had been training for this moment since I was 17. When the final bell sounded signalling the end of the fight, I knew I had won and the feeling was sublime. I was ecstatic about having my arm raised, announcing me the winner. The reason this was so important to me was that I did it alone and proved to myself that you can be master of your own destiny. I trained alone, I travelled to Japan alone, and I won alone. Being the only non-Japanese fighter and actually winning the All Japan Ju Jitsu Championship became a significant milestone in the ongoing development of my own martial arts doctrine.

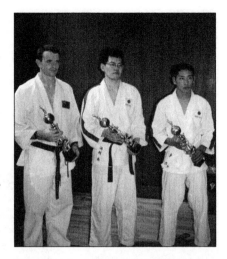

Heavyweight, middleweight and lightweight champions.

Chapter 9
Vancouver, Canada, 1998

Shortly after arriving back in Sydney from Japan in late July, I got an email from the International Sports Ju Jitsu (ISJA) President Ernie Boggs to see if I was sending an Australian team to the World Championships in Canada in November. At the time I was the ISJA Vice-President and the ISJA Australian Director, so I was planning on sending a team but was unsure at that stage whether I would compete or just coach the team.

For as long as I can remember I have been a bit of a worrier. It goes back to my childhood, when I was so unsure about what was happening with my parents. I had some minor panic attacks triggered by anxiety when I was 21, but up until the time I got back from my last trip to compete in Japan I had been pretty stable, mental health-wise.

But looking back now, there were signs earlier on that I was getting close to anxiety but I just brushed it off. There was no doubt that I was incredibly fatigued. I was working full time doing regular night shift as a flight attendant, running a small dojo, caring for a young family, renovating the house and competing. I was suffering from major burnout, but I just kept pushing.

I started to do a weird thing. I started to pay minute attention to normal body sensations I had not felt before, and literally started worrying about everything. I was later to learn that this was a classic symptom of general anxiety disorder. But at the time my doctor just prescribed a good night's sleep as I looked perfectly normal to him.

Poor chap. If only he knew how I really felt. In fact, outside of my immediate family no-one knew. On the surface I guess everything did look normal, but behind closed doors I had convinced myself I was dying. Back then I was no expert in anxiety, and the only advice I got from well-meaning people who knew me was to cheer up. Unfortunately, when you are in the grip of it those words make no sense at all.

So this is what I did. Instead of resting, regrouping and reducing stress, I decided the best thing for me was to load myself up and compete in another world championship.

Coming out and writing about this is difficult even now. What will people think of me? The stigma of strong men not being able to cope has plagued men for years, and in many cases has been – and still is – a silent killer. I did a great job of hiding it with my stoic, I'm-not-weak exterior while feeling the crushing weight of hopelessness on the inside.

During the months that followed I immersed myself in yoga to try and relax and reduce stress. I also started therapy. Both were great, as they started to release muscle tension and work on the source of the anxiety, which in turn opened me up to my deepest fears. The big one: you do not live forever. I realised I had a deep fear of dying, and my personal journey so far had been trying to come to terms with my own mortality.

This may seem obvious. But in the West we have a tendency to live in denial of death, not looking at it in any way until we have to. But this did not help me in any way. Realising I had a fear of dying was not the root of the problem. It was dying well that haunted me, again showing no weakness.

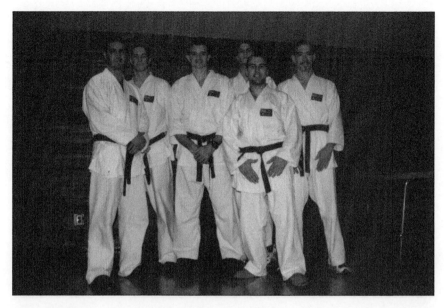

The strong ISJA Australian Team. L-R: Carl Safar, Dacian Moses, me, Steve Laurence, Norm Madden, Paul Henderson-Kelly.

So I continued portraying this tough impenetrable exterior as I ran a huge Ju Jitsu Championship in Sydney to choose a team to represent Australia. The tournament was a huge success, and we selected a great team. I would also compete and be the captain and coach. Looking back now, I don't know how I managed. I was still working as hard as ever.

The only thing that was beginning to change was an ever so slow, and I mean slow, feeling of peace around dying. It is very difficult to explain, as this is not something I can put into words. It was a feeling, a deeper understanding, that everything will be okay. So I continued on the path to Canada with this gentle awareness growing inside me that the experience in Canada was going to test me on so many levels. I have always chosen the most challenging path, and never make excuses for it being tough. But this time something was different. There was change in the air.

Ju jitsu is a Japanese martial art, so at previous world championships I felt they always lacked credibility because of the absence of a Japanese team. I was instrumental in introducing the ISJA Chairman Ernie Boggs to Aso Sensei, who then for the first time selected a Japanese team to compete in Canada. It was also great to see the inclusion of a Brazilian ju jitsu team

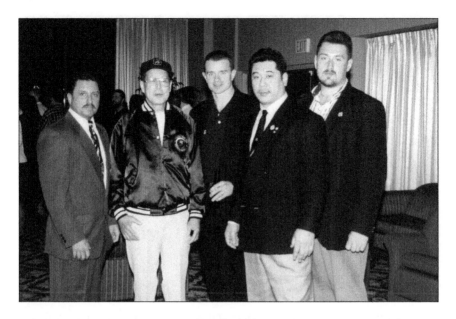

L–R: ISJA Chairman Ernie Boggs, American Ju Jitsu legend Wally Jay, Myself, Aso Sensei, USA Super Heavy Weight Champion Bob Steins.

for the first time. This was a true World Championships, and I was proud to have played a part in it all coming together. So in many ways I felt proud and that I had already won.

Arriving in Canada, I was still preoccupied with up-and-down waves of anxiety. But this was a huge event that needed my full attention, as the standard of competition was world class. Only five months had passed since competing in Japan. But unlike the Japanese competition, in Canada I felt like I was only just going through the motions, and surprised myself by lacking any real drive to win.

The tournament was overflowing with competitors and spectators from all over the world. On the outside I put on a brave face, but on the inside I was terrified. Would I be able to represent myself well and take the fight up to my opponents? Or would I crash and burn under the pressure of all that had happened over the past five months?

How was I going to hold it together and set an example to my fellow Australian team members, and not make a complete fool of myself in front of the entire Japanese team and other top competitors from around the world that I knew so well?

As fate would have it, the Australian team drew the British team in the first round of the team competition. Talk about getting thrown into the deep end. As the team captain my first fight was to be against English team captain and current World Heavyweight Champion, Gary Turner.

I remember how calm I was just chatting and exchanging pleasantries with Gary in the middle of the ring prior to the fight commencing. It seemed a world away from the war that was about to erupt between us. Gary and I had met several times before, but this was the first time we had met in the ring. I know he was keen to fight me, as he knew my reputation of being a hard and relentless competitor. My biggest fear was not losing. It was that I would not be able to match Gary and he would blow me off the floor. This feeling was new to me, as I have always given every fight I have been in my absolute all.

The fight started, and I was immediately drawn into its power. Regardless of how I was feeling, my body responded in the way it was trained. Gary fought a good fight, but I also landed some good shots and made him work for the win. I was happy I survived and exchanged blows with the best sports ju jitsu heavyweight in the world.

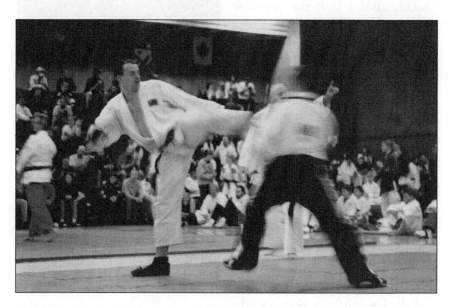

Standing toe to toe with Gary Turner in Canada. Gary was just too fast for me.

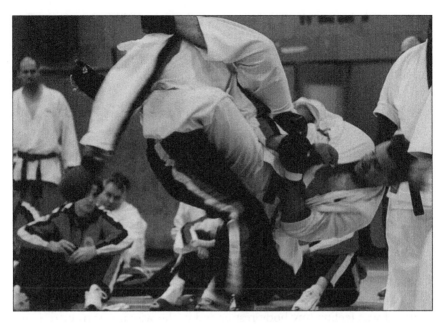

Attempting an arm lock on Gary. He just smiled at me.

I did not win any of my fights in Canada. But I won the personal struggle with myself. Regardless of the hesitation around my commitment to be a worthy competitor, and the extra stress caused by anxiety in the months beforehand, I was still able to keep it at bay and stand toe to toe with the best heavyweight sports ju jitsu fighters in the world.

The will to win may have finally been satisfied in my fight in Japan in July 1998. Going to Canada, I now realise, was necessary to farewell this part of my life. And what a way to do it. There has not been a world sports ju jitsu competition since that has had both the Japanese

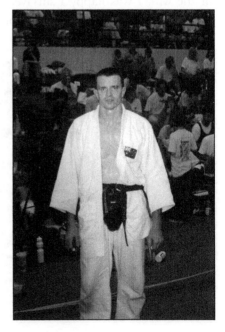

It is not about winning. It's all about doing your best.

and Brazilian teams attend, making this a truly authentic competition. As painful as this entire time was, I now felt free to continue my interest in martial arts as a vehicle of growth for body, mind and spirit. I was 35 and had been competing since I was 17 years old. I have never regretted retiring from competition.

Sparring as a path to enlightenment

After literally thousands of rounds of fighting and sparring, and frustrating myself for years by trying to take on and beat every martial arts student I could and going to extreme lengths to be the fastest, strongest and most powerful, I finally realised the real lesson.

I realised that winning and losing is totally irrelevant. There was something else that was driving me, and I now knew exactly what it was. I believe that during intense rounds of sparring you have to be so totally focused, calm, and in the present moment to survive. This can then lead to a clarity – a kind of oneness that can only be experienced when the movement of the mind very briefly stops.

In that space of stillness, when emotion rises and the mind moves, you can observe this process happen and not be affected by it. This exact process can be used in any interaction. By giving your full attention to the situation in front of you, and allowing presence and awareness to rise, you can be the witness to your emotions as they habitually rise and, in that brief moment, choose the correct response.

> *By learning to fight you no longer need to fight. I find this statement difficult. It took me years to get the desire to prove myself out of my system. I prefer to say that by learning to defend yourself you no longer feel the need to be aggressive.*

The last warrior

At the beginning of my martial arts journey I was training regularly with Master Tim Hassall, a taekwondo master, and black belts would often visit from other schools. It was not uncommon to see Tim sparring the visiting black belts before the commencement of the regular class. Back in those days there were no mats on the floors to cushion your training. It was all hard floor boards and bare feet. Personal protective equipment such as mouth guards and shin pads were rarely used. The training was rough, and had a military-like discipline. It was still quite rare to see women training in martial arts.

I remember one black belt in particular who used to regularly visit. His name was Graham Ball, and he was mid-height, not large, but a very intense fighter who pulled no punches. He snapped his kicks and punches through the air with deadly precision. He reminded me of Bruce Lee at his best. Though Tim was a great technician, he would be the first to agree with me that Graham probably would have better suited to something like the army special forces.

When I first sparred Graham I was still very new and inexperienced, and he hurt everything he touched. My forearms and shins were a mishmash of red lumps and large bruises, and although he scared me I respected him. We went on to spar many times, and he always managed to beat me up.

Over the years I trained with Tim Hassall, I sparred with many of the senior students. They did not care if you were a lower belt than them. They just wanted to win. There was one blue belt named Ron, and when I was a yellow belt he kicked towards my head and split me open between the eyes with the nail of his big toe. He was the first in line for me to train and beat. He got a real shock when I eventually bamboozled him with my kicks and punches.

I trained hard, and over the years eventually beat everyone in the class that had beaten me, including the black belts and eventually Tim himself.

Everyone except Graham Ball.

As I grew as a martial artist and won many competitions, it was always in the back of my mind that Graham was still out there and I feared him. I needed to find him and test myself. Not because he had wronged me, but because I deeply respected his ability. And to think I had finally been able to surpass him would be a huge milestone in my respect for my ability.

No matter how hard I looked for him, I just could not find him. There was no social media or Google back then, so all I could do was look in the White Pages telephone directory or check with people who knew him.

So I stopped looking. But I was always mindful that there remained one person out there somewhere that I feared.

It was some years later, when I had been working for Qantas for a couple of years, that I finally found Graham. I was in LA working at the time, and was walking towards the hotel lifts. I couldn't believe it. Graham Ball just walked right past me. He had not changed, and I recognised him in an instant. I stopped and called after him.

As it turned out we had been almost crossing paths for years, as he was also working for Qantas as a flight attendant. This was not strange, as there were 7000 flight attendants flying to different countries all over the world and you could go for years without bumping into friends. In 16 years of working for Qantas there were several crew in my original training class back in 1987 that I never saw again.

He remembered me immediately. This was too good to be true, so straight up I asked him if he wanted to train in the afternoon. He agreed, but suggested that before we spar we go on a bike ride first. I thought there would be no harm in that, and so agreed to do a ride on the beach boardwalk that runs from Redondo beach all the way to Santa Monica.

He tortured me on that bike ride. I should have known he would treat the bike ride like a life-or-death training session. We raced at every possible chance, Graham laughing over his shoulder as he well and truly sapped any remaining strength from my legs.

I finally made it back to the hotel and I was exhausted. Graham took one look at me and straight away suggested we go to the gym for sparring.

This was a perfect chance for him to take me out and he knew it. I knew I might not get another chance at this. To be honest the bike training did not phase me. The training I had already experienced in Korea, Thailand and Japan had fully prepared me for extreme training. I kind of overdid the looks of exhaustion and defeat, and Graham took the bait. I could not believe this was happening. I had dreamed of this chance for years. I was about to challenge myself against my toughest and most feared fighter.

From the moment we stood in front of each other to fight, I went into a very calm and still place. Totally present and at peace. I had trained for this for years. Graham started out by keeping his distance and feinting with moves to see how I reacted. I waited, maintaining poise, balance and awareness.

Without warning Graham launched everything at me, in an all-out attempt to take me down quickly. I simply avoided his kicks and punches and slipped out of his range. Easily spotting gaps in his defence, I placed my counter kicks and punches at ease, but without hurting him. I knew he was overwhelmed and had no answers to my movement. He put his hands down and walked away from me, completely lost and frustrated at not being able to land even a finger on me. I had done this without hurting him. This was the perfect outcome. There were no hard feelings, and we remained friends for many years.

What separates a great black belt from a good black belt is their ability to use the exact amount of force necessary. Nothing more, nothing less.

When you finally get to a place where you can beat your opponent without touching or hurting them, you are getting close to mastery. Giving and compassion are just as important as fighting and hurting. The true warrior needs to understand they are as important as each other, but the basic warrior philosophy should always be to choose peace.

The next level of black belt, Japan, 2008

Each time I go back to Japan to train in Daito Ryu, my old friend fear meets me as soon as I get off the aircraft. Knowing what is coming up, it's no wonder I just want to turn around and go straight home. But my body keeps moving in the direction of the dojo, regardless of the constantly rotating thoughts on why this can't be good for me. Before I know it, I am in my uniform and bowing as I enter the dojo. *No turning back now.*

Though I had retired from competition, I still continued to grade and move up the black belt ranks in several martial arts. It had been 12 years since my initial grading to black belt in Daito Ryu. I arrived in Tokyo late on Friday evening and got the train directly to Shinkoiwa, which is about an hour towards Tokyo from Narita airport. It's an industrial type area, not pretty in any way and well away from the action in Tokyo central.

I checked into my hotel and crashed in the tiny room after the long flight. I spent all day Saturday visiting some of my favourite spots in Tokyo – the Kinokuniya bookshop, relaxing in Shinjuku Park, eating lunch of sushi and fresh sashimi, and picking up my favourite rice crackers and sweets.

Though I was trying to distance myself from the emotional attachment of grading and working hard to stay calm, fear and trepidation were constant companions sharing the moment.

At the grading you never know what Sensei is going to put you through. Though I had fully prepared, I just knew he was going to test me on something that was beyond my preparation. I checked out of my room on Sunday morning and walked the 20 minutes to the dojo. As I turned the last corner and saw the dojo building, I was overwhelmed with a feeling of wanting to run as fast as I could in the opposite direction.

Yet my body kept moving closer and closer.

Fear and dread started to rise within. This is where my years of training kicked in. I was able to allow whatever emotion or feeling came forward then and watch it as an observer – not letting it get a hold of me, not becoming the emotion. So I could still see clearly what needed to be done and just get on with it.

I believe this is one of my 'secrets of success', and has enabled me to navigate successfully through fears and other stuff that can cripple and stop you from getting where you want to be.

I met Sensei in his office on the second floor of the building that housed his construction company and the dojo on the third floor, and I gave him a bottle of good Aussie wine. (Not a bribe, just a nice custom.) It was great to see the dojo again. It is quite small but quite beautiful. The walls are adorned with calligraphy by the famous swordsman and Tesshu, Admiral Takeshi, who was one of the original founder's most famous students, and Aikido's Ueshiba Sensei. All priceless.

As I stepped onto the dojo floor I instantly remembered the quality of the mats – hard and unforgiving. There was no room for error today.

Sensei said he had organised for a team of students to come in and assist with the grading. Merek from Poland was to be my main partner and take the bulk of the throws. So as he entered the dojo wearing only a white belt I was somewhat alarmed. Everyone else who takes this kind of test has a partner of the same rank or higher, and is at least a black belt.

This is important because the partner must know how to fall in order to be safe. It makes the process much more efficient and safe, and you can demonstrate the moves without fear of injuring your partner. Merek did not know what the moves were. He did not even know what to attack with. I started to get worried. I had 60 moves to demonstrate with precision and accuracy, and my partner did not have a clue.

My balance had been broken and I was starting to panic. *Stay calm, Andy. Don't let your fears show. Just do your best with what you have been given* became my mantra.

So for the first hour I really struggled. I was instructing a beginner on how to attack and receive very dangerous moves, and at the same time trying my hardest not to hurt him as I locked, choked and threw him. Sensei kept saying over and over, 'Andy, no good. Andy, no good'.

My confidence was being sapped and failure loomed. But I just kept on going.

An hour into the session, four fresh white belts arrived. All four were Japanese Aikido 4th Dan Black Belts, but still white belts in Daito Ryu so they also did not have a clue on what techniques were needed. But they were fresh and full of beans, ready to test me out.

Sensei came up to me and said, 'Andy, today I just watch. No time for grading'.

I was in shock. All this preparation, time and money, and he was not even going to grade me. I looked up at the clock and thought, *That's it. Time to leave.* But I didn't. I just thought, *Don't show what is going on inside. Be neutral. No matter what just do the technique, let go of the need to have an outcome, just enjoy the experience. You now have no need to prove anything.*

I decided I was going to do the techniques as best and as hard as I could while still looking after my partners. I hit out hard in each move, my focus and awareness were intense, and I could feel my partners' fear. All the preparation, years of it, played its part in helping me remain composed and in control.

Sensei would make me repeat moves time and time again. 'No, no, no. That's bad. That's not right,' he would yell at me, then look at me with disgust and say, 'Wakaru ka?' ('Do you get it?'). My response would always be, 'Hai wakarimashita' ('Yes sir, I understand') as I bowed deeply.

This went on for three hours, much later than I expected. It was getting close to the deadline for my train back to the airport. I had taught, and responded to the required moves for my belt level, so there was no reason to stay. As I bowed and asked politely for permission to leave I felt extremely disappointed and lost, but was happy I had done everything that was asked of me well.

As I entered the change room, Sensei came up to me and said, 'Andy, bring your clothes and get changed downstairs in my office'. As I entered his office he presented me with my 2nd Dan certificate in Daito Ryu Aiki ju jitsu. He made a point of telling me that my technique was very bad, but I passed. I was confused, but elated.

I did not have time to think about the process too much as I sprinted for a taxi to get my train on time. I went directly from the dojo to Narita airport, checked in, and flew home.

Sensei knew I would be well prepared. After 20 years he knows me well, and has seen me in action many times. This grading really tested me on many levels. It became a test of my spirit. He broke me down to the level of beginner and watched to see how I would respond. It was a great test for me. I had to completely let go of every identification and expectation and just keep moving ahead moment by moment, technique by technique. If I did not do this, I would have 'lost it' early in the day.

When the path has a beginning and an end, the journey may start and finish with an end point in mind. The past and future becomes the focus. Where the way has no start and no end, the journey becomes the focus. Each step, each breath, each moment.

Chapter 10
Power talk

From 1992 until 1998 I was travelling and training a lot overseas, and I used the opportunity to interview top martial arts exponents and write a column for a popular Australian martial arts magazine. This was a great opportunity to get inside knowledge, ask questions that could directly influence my own personal journey, and get access to people who wouldn't ordinarily be as easy to talk to.

Though I did not follow a particular pattern for selecting people to interview, I had one criterion for choosing: they had to be excelling in their chosen pursuit of martial arts. I hoped that by interviewing world leaders in martial arts it would take me closer to finding that one true master who exuded the qualities of excellence in all aspects of body, mind and spirit.

All of my interview subjects were so diverse. No story was the same. Each had to endure and overcome incredible hardship and challenges to reach and maintain their level of excellence. The following are just a few of the masters I had the privilege to meet. What follows is not the interview but my own commentary on details about each experience.

The Locomotive, Tokyo, 1993

Tokyo, still the martial arts Mecca of the world. Not outwardly visible, but in just about every school and gym throughout this vast metropolis the martial arts still play a huge part in the daily lives of many Japanese men, women and children. For the uninitiated, non-speaking foreigner, the task of finding a suitable martial arts school is definitely no easy one.

For most of the popular styles that have their main headquarters in Tokyo, finding and entering these schools is no real problem. They have English speaking staff, and quite often foreigners actually work at the school. But these popular schools can be so overrun with people from all over the globe that they actually have foreigner classes. You end up not even training with the Japanese, so there is no real difference between the Japanese school and your own school at home.

The whole Japanese training experience does not just start when you bow in at the beginning of class. In fact, by the time you reach your school you have probably already been working out for an hour battling the massive crowds at Shinjuku or Ikebukero station, jostling and hustling just to get on the train, let alone get a seat. And you can expect worse crowds on the way home. Or do they just seem worse because you are tired?

Anyway, unless you are wearing earphones and have your eyes closed, be prepared to become 'Instant English Teacher' and politely nod your head in agreement as the drunk businessman beside you battles around the 'L's and R's' of the English language while you nimbly duck and weave the stench of his tobacco- and sake-smelling breath.

But don't despair. For those interested people who would prefer to venture a little deeper, there are a multitude of lesser-known schools more than eager to let you train. At these schools you may find yourself being the only foreigner, but at least you know you are getting the real deal and not second-hand teachings from another foreigner.

There is one such school tucked deep in the centre of Tokyo. It is a small but very serious karate dojo. Upon entering this particular dojo you can feel there is something different about it. There are no wall-to-wall trophies or colour posters of the instructor. Just a simple shrine and the rules of the dojo written underneath it. To the left as you walk in is a small weights area, and to the right you'll see various well-used pads and punching bags so characteristic of a full-contact dojo. But this is no ordinary full-contact dojo, and it is definitely not for the faint-hearted.

The style is Daido Juku, and the Sensei Takashi Azuma. Azuma Sensei has done what no other instructor has dared to do. He has taken Kyokushin that little bit further by adding the punching, knees and elbows of Thai boxing and the throwing, grappling and

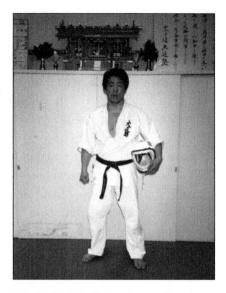

Head of Daido Juku, Azuma Sensei.

ground work of judo and wrestling, and then taken away the boxing gloves and replaced them with mitts smaller than punching bag mitts.

Azuma Sensei has an impressive karate history. After battling through two World Kyokushin Championships and numerous All Japan Championships, he finally took first place in the 1979 All Japan Kyokushin Championships. During his tournament fighting years Azuma Sensei was nicknamed 'The human locomotive' because of his steam train approach to fighting and heavy use of low kicks and throwing techniques.

After winning the All Japan Championships, Azuma Sensei became disillusioned with the methods and limitations of one karate style, and so took the initiative and decided to venture out alone. Since that time Daido Juku has grown considerably.

With 56 dojos and some 10,000 students, it is famous throughout Japan for its hard and effective fighting system. Azuma Sensei stresses reality in martial arts, and so the students are well disciplined in all fighting ranges, moving easily from the kicking and punching range to the grappling and ground work range. The training sessions are varied and well structured, with different instructors emphasising the techniques according to the lesson format.

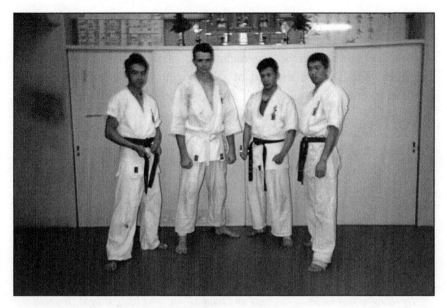

Standing with Daido Juku senior students.

The classes are not designed to be fun. There is always an air of seriousness and intensity throughout the lesson. The sparring sessions are a real test of one's fighting skills. You're in there boots and all, with groin kicking, joint attacks and head butts the norm. After a few sessions of sparring you really know whether your previous training has prepared you adequately for a street encounter.

I first trained at Azuma Sensei's Tokyo Daido Juku Dojo in 1991 to get a feel for the style. After a couple of sessions, Azuma Sensei invited me to spar him. I took this as a great honour, although I was quite afraid as he had an awesome reputation. The sparring match was a torrid affair, the contact getting heavier and heavier the longer it went on.

I lifted my left leg to throw my signature (and at times very effective) high turning kick, and Sensei immediately kicked my support right leg out from under me. I came down hard, crashing into the weights area next to the dojo. Sensei did not stop. He jumped straight on top of me but I was too quick, taking him to side control. I was working hard for an arm submission, but he was too strong.

We stood up, and Sensei launched himself back at me. He oozed intensity, and kept the pressure on as we continued to trade blows. It was easy to see and feel the reason he was nicknamed 'The human locomotive' by his peers. Sensei called the end of the fight, and his killer-like intensity changed to one of mutual respect as he smiled and said, 'Good fight'.

Azuma Sensei is still a class fighter who is definitely unique in his approach to fighting. But fighting, he says, is not the end result of training. And Budo is one of the many ways to educate young people, hopefully guiding them along an honest and moral road where they can develop into outstanding members of the community. This attitude is reflected by his many black belts who are all courteous, humble and well educated. Most of them hold jobs as businessmen, and still enjoy the realistic, rough-and-tumble training of Daido Juku Karate.

By choosing non-violence, kindness and compassion, your being is light. You will go for years without ever having to raise your voice.

National Japanese treasure

Otake Sensei is head teacher of the famous Japanese martial arts school, the Katori Shinto Ryu. He is one of the greatest swordsman of the modern era, and holds the auspicious honour of being named a living Japanese national treasure. It took quite a lot of communication back and forth between Otake Sensei and my then wife Hisako to secure this interview. In fact, had it not been for Hisako's understanding of the correct Japanese etiquette there is no way Otake Sensei would have spoken to me.

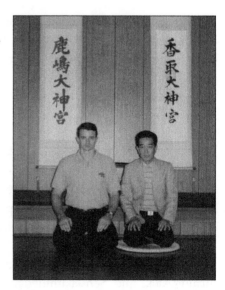

Sitting with Otake Sensei.

Arriving at his Narita residence, which is in a farming town about one hour out of Tokyo by fast train, we were warmly welcomed by Otake Sensei. He seemed especially impressed that I had brought Hisako with me. Which was prudent, as my Japanese was not good enough to understand the details of the explanation by Otake Sensei.

We went through the interview, and he was entertaining and animated with his explanations. As the answers were quite detailed, it was some months before I could get them translated and fully appreciate the time this great master had given me. He shared an incredible insight into the ways and rites of this highly traditional way of the samurai.

There are very few true classical Japanese martial arts masters still alive. I mean masters of martial arts that were developed on the battlefield and have remained unchanged to the present. Fighting arts whose masters were the last of the true warrior class. Within 10 years all of the famous pre-war masters will have passed away. With their passing most will take their secrets, and their arts will simply disappear.

In Japan, the classical martial arts dojos can be hard to find. And it is no wonder. The masters retreat into their dojos out of fear they will be aligned with Mutant Ninja Turtles, Power Rangers, Mortal Combat or any number of other shows/movies that continue to misinterpret martial arts. They close their doors, and no amount of money will get them open again.

In their place will remain the myriad of hybrid forms, most void of any real substance. Yet the student, with nothing to compare it with, is deluded into thinking his/her art is true martial arts. All the supercilious floss that so many attach to the martial arts only serves to fill the gaping hole created by a severe lack of knowledge. Would the modern dojo survive without the multi-coloured, embroidered, badge-covered uniforms, the glint of the chrome-covered plastic trophies, carpet and mirrored walls, and the empty promises of becoming superhuman?

Katori Shinto Ryu is classical martial art. It is as it should be: plain, no frills and real. This dojo is not concerned with petty skirmishes that resemble two seagulls squabbling over a chip. Their training is simple: you learn to cut, and you learn to kill. But with this knowledge comes responsibility, for since the beginning of this martial art the warrior, if allowed to choose, always chose peace over war.

Not just anyone can enter the Katori Shinto Ryu. All applicants are carefully screened, and many are turned away. Those who are accepted sign their signature with blood, and are expected to train diligently without question. There is no such thing as 'freestyling' or modernising the techniques. They are done as they have always been done, and will continue to be done.

Students do not enter Katori to learn self-defence. Many have already spent years perfecting other martial arts. Students are taught a complete martial art system – Kenjutsu (sword cutting), Naginata (spear), Iaijutsu (sword drawing), Ju Jitsu (self-defence), and many more skills. The timber floors are hard, and the walls are bare. There is no air-conditioning in summer, and no heating in winter. The training is in pairs, fast and furious. One slip or lapse of concentration with the Bokken would mean serious injury.

Otake Sensei is not only a martial arts warrior but also a spiritual one. To be a spiritual warrior means to develop a special kind of courage, one that is innately intelligent, gentle and fearless. He is the keeper of the style, and it is his responsibility to ensure the art continues in its original form into the next century.

I have included four key points of Otake Sensei's interview that I found inspirational.

> *To temper the ego, the martial artist must do physical and spiritual training. By doing so it reduces the ego, allowing the true exponent to celebrate happiness and joy with others and feel sorrow from the heart. This is true martial art. But this is also the most difficult path. Confrontation of self, an egoless path, is so removed from modern martial arts practice. Yet through the ages the true warriors were not concerned with external shows of strength. Their trophy was life itself. I hear the word 'warrior' used so often these days, but these people have no idea.*

> *Choisai Sensei, the founder of Katori Shinto Ryu, lived by three rules. For the individual continually striving to improve, polish your technique and polish every aspect of your life, mentally, spiritually and physically. Strive to improve even when your body craves rest and sleep. Avoid bad mouthing others and creating a grudge. Commit to a peaceful life.*

> *Humans should strive to become rounded both mentally and physically. If you are square and have acute angles, metaphorically speaking you are always hitting and bumping people both mentally and physically. If you have angles you catch other people. Being round enables you to bump off, glide past.*

> *If you pull a square piece of board through a shallow clear pond the corners will continually catch the bottom, churning up the water and creating rough, dirty and choppy water. If the board is round it is okay. You can pull it through easily. People are the same. They have to become rounded. It is the path of least resistance.*

A final note

Weeks later I arrived back at his dojo, camera in hand. I asked for permission to take some class photos and without answering my question, Sensei abruptly asked where my wife was. I told him that unfortunately she couldn't make it. He just grunted, turned away from me, and did not speak to me again. I quickly took some photos and excused myself, feeling quite unpopular. I was quite shocked at the difference in his demeanour. But knew I had a good story.

Fighting Judo Gene, Los Angeles, December 1994

There are flashes of pink as the crowd shifts. I can hear his voice, the twang of the American drawl, but I still cannot see him. The crowd parts in preparation for the training session and Gene heads towards me, a mass of double-woven pink judo uniform and a mat of red hair. Expecting a loudmouthed self-adulating braggart, I brace myself in anticipation of an egocentric verbal assault reminiscent of so many champions in the martial arts, but even more so from the man nicknamed by so many of his peers as 'The toughest fighter in the world'.

I should have learnt by now to always expect the unexpected. It never ceases to amaze me how first impressions can be so wrong. Gene immediately puts me at ease by his unassuming and gentle nature.

Squeezing the last of any life out of my hand, he welcomes me like a long-lost brother. This man is impressive, but not just in the physical sense. He does not need words, as his presence carries his message.

Gene is generous with his time. After 40 years in martial arts the love affair is still as strong as ever. But don't let him grab you and avoid his stare. And whatever you do, do not volunteer to help him demonstrate a move. World champion kickboxer and karate legend Bennie the Jet was right when he said Gene is the best fighter he has trained with. He will crank the choke on your neck and sing a lullaby while your body shakes, convulses and unconsciously revolts against the impending sleep.

Gene says choking someone out is not what injures people. It's when he lets them go and they hit the ground. He throws a few one-liners, and eyes the group for another volunteer (or should I say victim). While I edge my

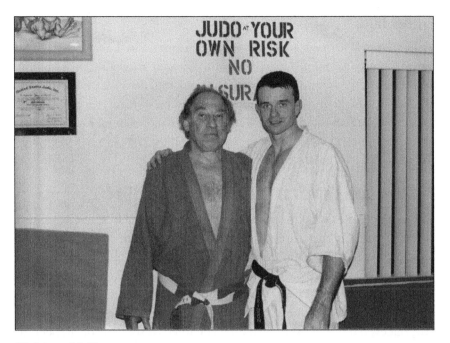

Training with Gene.

way to the back of the room the other seminar attendees jump in line like children waiting for a rollercoaster ride, strangely eager for their turn to be choked out by the great Gene Le Bell.

Gene Le Bell is one of the great grandmasters of martial arts in America. Friend and training partner of the late Bruce Lee, grappling instructor of world-renowned martial arts legends Bennie the Jet, Bill Wallace and the late Joe Lewis, and mentor and friend to other great martial artists too numerous to name. Yet there are no airs or graces. He is simply a man still confident in his ability intent on spreading his legacy to anyone who is willing to learn.

I asked Gene about Bruce Lee, and this is what he had to say.

> *The first time I was on the set of his TV show* The Green Hornet *he was the driver 'Kato'. And he did this new karate-like martial art called kung fu. He was very standoffish, very dignified and very classy. So I picked him up and ran down the set with him over my shoulder. He weighed 130lbs and I weighed*

about 190lbs. He said, 'Don't do that'. He would get in a kung fu pose, and I would pick him up and run back the other way.

He was extremely good. I went to his martial arts school, and we would share techniques. Then he would come down to my place and we would work out in the afternoon with nobody around. I believe I was the one who actually got him to raise his hands like a boxer. They used to be right down here [indicating hands at the waist], and then he started to hold his hands up in the later movies. He was a great, great showman.

Brandon Lee, his son, was also a stuntman and a great kung fu man. He brought Brandon down to the set, and he was good. I thought he was better than his father Bruce Lee.

Bruce Lee loved to grapple. You know, play around on the ground. But he said it won't sell movies, and he was right. People were not ready for it. The action was in standing fighting.

He was telling me about John Wayne. He said, 'Look at this. All the fighting that he does is standing. You get knocked down and you jump back up and he does something else. That is what people want to see. Something moving around standing up. It might change. Everything in life goes through fads'.

I never had any altercations with Bruce. In fact, I used to take the falls that he liked. I used to take the high martial arts falls, and although I didn't work in any movies with him I did work some in TV shows with him.

We then had a bit of a Q&A session.

Me: *And what do you attribute to your success?*

Gene: *Well, first of all, it helps if you are a fanatic. If you are a fanatic, you are going to work that much harder. Now I am not as coordinated as a lot of people, and truly not as smart. I am certainly better looking than any of my opponents, so I have got to work out harder than everybody else...*

Me: *And that fanaticism turns into total commitment?*

Gene: Yes, total, total commitment. And when you work, you have got to be so good that it is second nature. When I am wrestling, I don't say I am going for a top wrist lock or a short arm scissors or a figure four double ouch. I go to the closest thing to me and grab it, and if I miss it I go to the next thing.

The world's largest fighter, Tokyo, September 1994

"That's what sumo was to me at that time – proving people wrong. That's the thing that got me fired up. People were saying I ain't going to make it, that no-one else is going to make it after Takoniyama, so I proved them wrong." – Konishiki

Even as I walked through the main entrance of the three-storey building of the Takeshiabeya dojo, I was still uncertain as to whether this interview would take place. The Japanese Sumo Association is a very closed-door group that protects the best interests of its sumo wrestlers with a guarded fervour.

Although they gave a 'Yes' on behalf of Konishiki (sumo wrestlers are given a Japanese name), the decision was still up to him on the day. It is difficult for even locals to get close to the sumo stars, who are amongst the most popular sporting stars in Japan. But perseverance eventually paid off, and at least I made it inside the front door.

We were met at the front entrance, a small doorway that seemed ambiguous to a building that is the home of so many large men. To the left of the door were beer and sake stacked to the ceiling. Sumo must be the only sport where drinking is encouraged to excess.

The man who meets us has no idea about any interview, and waves us into a room that looks over the training area. Sitting on the hard tatami mats waiting, I watch the young apprentice sumos go through the last stages of their morning workout. They are the new blood, scouted from high schools all over Japan. Right now they are at the absolute bottom rank of Sumo, the toilet-cleaning wall scrubbers who must attend to every need of their senior ranks.

Naked except for their obi (belt), they are all rotund though proud of their size. They remind me of large cuddly babies rolling in a sand pit. But there is one difference. They all proudly wear the top knot, the symbol of the samurai outlawed at the turn of the 20th century. The sumo are the only

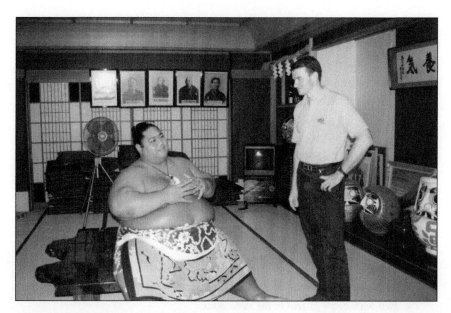

Sumo giant, Konishiki. I found him to exude warmth. He is charismatic and honest in his love for the Japanese people, and for his sport.

men in Japan allowed to display it. The top knot has great significance, for like the samurai the world of sumo is governed by strict discipline and etiquette. It is part of the classic Japanese culture, a symbol of an era passed and one of the last bastions of a culture almost completely seduced by the West.

The Japanese are very proud of sumo and keep it well guarded. They fear that sumo, like so many other aspects of their martial arts culture, will fall victim to time and end up resembling no more than a comical display of brute strength and steroid-induced anger with no significance, similar to professional wrestling.

There are no special concessions for foreigners entering into this world. They must toe the line like all new wrestlers. Many come, but few make it.

Konishiki, originally from Samoa, came and made his presence felt immediately. At 190cm tall and 280kg in weight Konishiki is massive, though not just in body size. His popularity now fans well beyond the shores of Japan. His mountain-like frame has appeared in magazines and newspapers around the world.

He had a meteoric rise through the lower ranks and burst into the champion Makushita division, taking on and defeating all who got in his way. He rose to the champion rank of Ozeki, the highest rank ever achieved by a foreign wrestler, and remained there for some time, paving the way for acceptance of foreigners into this most Japanese of Japanese cultural sports.

Talking with him was easy. He was very humble, and did not make a big thing out of the tough lifestyle. The highly popular Konishiki said he yearned for a normal life, and was looking forward to the day when he could do normal family things such as take his kids to Disneyland without people noticing him. I thought that was very funny, considering his fame and size.

Everything starts from stillness and finishes with stillness. In fact, stillness is the constant from where everything arises. Go from zero to 100% in the blink of an eye, then back down to zero in the same blink.

Aikido master, Zen priest, Los Angeles, 5 July 1994

Right in the middle of downtown LA, just two blocks past Little Tokyo tucked away in a row of warehouses, is a magnificently re-created Japanese martial arts dojo.

The only giveaway that East meets West in this old rail warehouse is the mass of bamboo that lines the front wall. As you step over the threshold to the entrance, the hum of LA drops away behind you and are met by the serene and airy interior of an authentic Japanese martial arts dojo.

Everything about it is Japanese. It was even created using Japanese timber by Japanese craftsmen. It is hard to believe that this dojo is in the middle of downtown LA. It doesn't quite seem to fit the mould of other American martial arts schools. Where are the stars-and-stripes boxing gloves and martial arts uniforms? And where are all the trophies?

But then again, the instructor is as unique as the dojo he created. Reverend Kensho Furuya began his study of Aikido in 1961. He received a university grant and completed a degree in Asian Studies, trained at the Aikido World Headquarters in Tokyo under Kisshomaru Ueshiba Sensei, attended Harvard, began his own school teaching in Hollywood, began a column called 'Ancient Way' for *Martial Training* magazine, was President

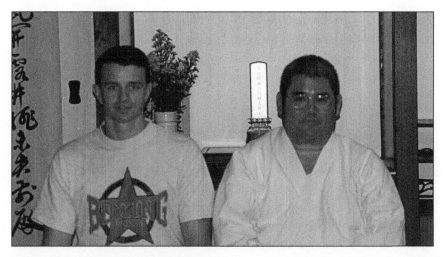

With Reverend Kensho Furuya Sensei.

of the Southern Californian Sword Society, established the first official branch school of the All Japan Batto Do Federation, became an ordained Zen priest under Bishop Kenko Yamashita of the Soto Zen Buddhism Sect, and accompanied Bishop Yamashita to speak at the United Nations in New York.

And for the past 12 years, as well as writing for various magazines and working on several books, he has been running The Aikido Centre of Los Angeles full time.

Furuya Sensei himself was warm and welcoming. It was Christmas Eve, so things were quiet everywhere. Being a Buddhist monk, I was unsure if he celebrated Christmas.

I was initially surprised by his size, as he was quite a large man. I tried not think about it as I commenced the interview. I was keen to see how Sensei integrated his martial arts and spirituality.

We spoke for more than an hour and, as usual, if you ask the right questions the information will flow. I was impressed with the simplicity of his philosophy and his in-depth analysis and understanding of Aikido and its place in modern society. Sensei has integrated his martial arts seamlessly with the Zen religion. He has not overdone it either way, and can relate the lessons of both Aikido and Zen in a way that makes sense.

But after the tape stopped he let loose with a tirade of profanity. After the interview finished, he asked me what I was up to next. Being Christmas Eve, he invited me to join him for lunch. I was being picked up by my mate Mark Sumi, and we were off to meet a very well-known Daito Ryu practitioner Don Angier. I mentioned this to Sensei and I was shocked by his response.

We had just spent the past hour delving into the depths of martial arts and personal growth. So I was surprised by such judgement from someone who has done so much Aikido (which is the art of peace), and the time he has spent in meditation. But I quickly reminded myself of the frailty of the human psyche and the power of habitual ways of thinking. So luckily, because of the work I had done on myself, from my own perspective I did not judge or criticise him. I just made a mental note again to not expect mastery from so-called masters.

I was sad to hear of Furuya Sensei's sudden death in March 2007. He was a well-respected master who had taught and influenced thousands of lives.

He died of a heart attack while teaching at his beloved dojo.

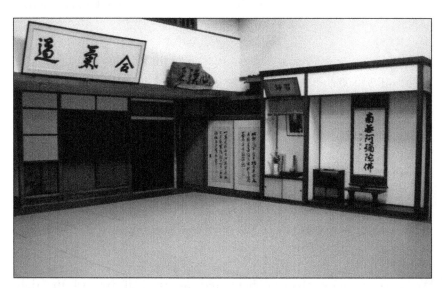

Furuya Sensei recreated a beautiful Japanese dojo in downtown LA.

Chapter 11
The incredible Taebo

I n the late 90s there was an incredible boom in cardio martial arts. It was the latest fitness fad, and it swept the world. American karate legend Billy Blanks took his taekwondo skills and added them to aerobic sequences, added in the latest music, and created Taebo. It was huge. Billy recorded Taebo and made millions selling the DVDs through television. I visited his gym and Taebo headquarters, and was stunned by the number of people who were there for the 10am class – well over 100. And classes went from 6am until 10pm. Experiencing the Taebo class was very hard, and it was a challenge to complete the entire class.

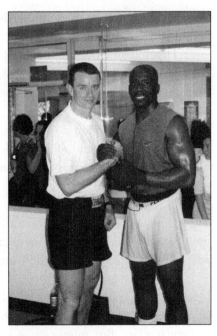

The inspirational Billy Blanks.

I was lucky to be able to interview Billy and gain some incredible insights into how and why he put the Taebo program together. Billy was humble, and spoke with an honest certainty. He is deeply spiritual, and bases his success on his faith. He will take any opportunity to espouse his beliefs, often using the vehicle of his class formats to preach the gospel. Did I think this was too much? No. It was no different to Reverend Furuya and his Buddhist teachings, or Otake Sensei and the Shinto religion. The thing about Billy Blanks was that he really believed and lived his modern interpretation of martial arts and spirituality. It was refreshing, and after sitting down and talking with him I would say he is the closest to being a true master that I have met on my travels.

The Aiki ju jitsu master

I had the privilege of being close to Katsuyuki Kondo Sensei, one of the greatest ju jitsu masters of the modern era. The connection lasted 25 years. I have already written extensively about my experiences at Daito Ryu Aiki Ju Jitsu, but there was ultimately one defining moment at the Sensei's dojo in Japan that was to change my outlook and the course of my training.

When I first started training under Kondo Sensei he was one scary dude. Not in an angry or aggressive way. It was more his powerful energy and life force. His charisma was intense. Sensei was committed to the dissemination of the correct method of Daito Ryu, or rather his interpretation of what was taught to him mainly by the founder's son Takeda Tokimune.

Sensei saw that the key to the long-term survival of his art was in the teaching of foreigners. So, when I was living in Japan in 1991, every Sunday my brother John, Mark Sumi and I would go to Sensei's dojo for special training.

These private classes would start at 10am. We would train until 12, and then Sensei would treat us to an amazing Japanese lunch prepared by his wife. We would then train again from 1pm until 4pm.

I cherish those training sessions and the time Sensei put into training us. He showed many techniques and variations of techniques that were not taught in regular class. But mostly these training sessions were just a continual repetition of the basics. 'Again, again,' Sensei would repeat like a mantra. We drilled the moves for hours, until the basics became second nature.

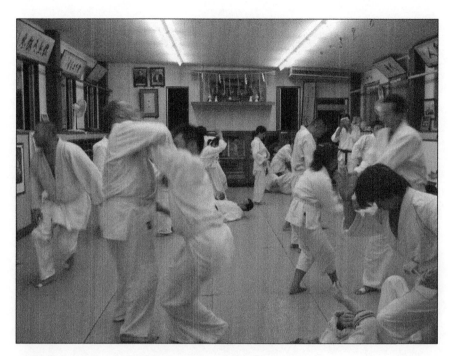

Training at the Daito Ryu Headquarters. Tokyo Japan.

Instead of using the air conditioner Sensei would just open all the windows, hoping for a cool breeze. But the air was always so thick and still. Every now and then a moth would land on the tatami mats amidst the crashing bodies. Sensei would stop the class immediately and rescue the helpless moth. This tiny creature struggling for life amidst these falling giants was given a reprieve by the kindness of this great ju jitsu master, who exemplified the essence of his art by gently rescuing the moth.

I value every moment of my time spent under the tutelage of Kondo Sensei, and he would often say martial arts and life are one. But how martial arts and life were one to him, and how he accomplished that, he kept to himself. Like all the masters I have met, trained under and experienced, he could not separate himself from his sense of self-importance long enough to be considerate to the path of his students. He was also subject to the frailties of the ego.

From 1988 up until August 2013 I was a loyal and dedicated student of Kondo Sensei and his Daito Ryu lineage, eventually grading to 2nd Dan black belt. I officially resigned from Daito Ryu and Kondo Sensei after

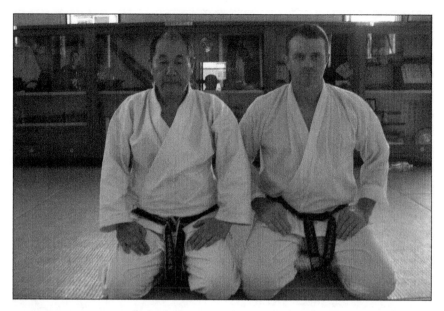

One of my last photos with Kondo Sensei.

one of my senior students undermined my relationship with Sensei. They brought him out to Sydney to visit, and applied – and was accepted to open – a Daito Ryu study group in Sydney. I was shocked and disappointed, but I still arranged to meet him and his wife for lunch. Sensei was short and unfriendly, and lunch was very uncomfortable. It was clear that whatever the senior student had said to Kondo Sensei meant our friendship was over.

Apparently, loyalty and honour only apply to martial arts when it is convenient. Hence I resigned, as I no longer had trust or faith in the integrity of my teacher or his new branch in Australia. My name was subsequently emblazoned across the Daito Ryu website home page, banning me from learning or teaching Daito Ryu.

In April 2017 I sent an email, not to try and re-enter Kondo Sensei's dojo but to heal old wounds. It was cathartic for me, as I was able to see my part in it all and apologise for any hurt I may have caused. Forgiveness is a quality I admire, and as I did not hear back I assumed that any forgiveness was beyond this great master.

By conducting these interviews, I was not looking to learn a superior way of fighting. I was keen to see if they had gone beyond the desire to be the best, and to see if there was more to them than just their physical techniques. Had they gone beyond just being a dojo martial artist and created a philosophy on mastery by which they lived their everyday life? And how willing were they to share it?

I soon came to realise that none of these so-called masters could give me any real insights into how they integrated (if they did at all) their teachings into a philosophy to live by. Was I expecting too much? We are all human, and unless we take the training, be it meditation, therapy or something else, to understand the inner workings of our mind, we will always be a slave to desires, habits and destructive ways of thinking that even the masters are not exempt from.

The men I interviewed were all fine men, and have been an incredible influence on thousands of students worldwide. They all represent martial arts to the best of their ability. Unfortunately, for me this was not enough.

After conducting the interviews, and together with my own experiences, I began to understand that there are many paths that lead up the mountain to mastery. And no matter how high we climb, there is always a higher mountain. Mastery is not perfection. Mastery is the attainment of wisdom.

The master

From the age of 17 until I left my job as a flight attendant, I kicked and punched my way around the world, going from fight to fight, dojo to dojo, country to country, grading to competition to seminar, driven at first by deep insecurities from my childhood and teens. At the same time I was looking for the master teacher who could jet-propel me to become an all-knowing spiritual warrior and guide me to a deeper understanding of myself.

The entire time I was looking outside of myself for someone else to give me all the answers. But the time was never wasted, as I feel it was all necessary for me to go through in order to prepare me for the next stage of my journey.

By the time I finally left my job as a flight attendant in 2003 I had kicked, punched and wrestled myself to a standstill. I no longer had the desire to seek new challenges, and was satisfied that I no longer had anything to prove to myself about who or what I was. I could finally stand with my head held high in the knowledge that I did my absolute best in all challenges that I was faced with. I would not change a thing.

At about the same time as I left my job I found meditation again, or rather it found me. Meditation has been a constant in my life ever since, and over the past 15 years I have come to realise that it has added a much-needed dimension to my martial arts and to my life. By turning my attention inward, I have been able to enhance my sense of awareness of who I am and what makes me tick, and gain a far deeper awareness of others.

I am no longer angry or impatient, and I can sit in stillness through most conflict. I don't react spontaneously as I used to. There is a clear space allowing me to choose an appropriate response to the true needs of any situation. I attribute this wisdom firstly to the 25 years needed to extinguish the burning desire to seek wisdom and knowledge outside of myself.

Plenty of doors would open for me, but the rooms were always empty. Finally, I found what I call my door marked 'Summer'. The door into my higher self. An inner knowing and light that illuminates the path of the spiritual warrior, free from past experiences that had controlled me. Through this door was peace and happiness in the present moment. I opened the door and finally found the master I had been looking for, and he had been here the whole time.

This door opens to incredible options when you believe in your own inner master.

The years looking for the master outside of myself finally led to the realisation that only the inward journey is true mastery.

It took me years to understand this. But I would not have come to this point unless I'd had all these experiences. The journey led me back to the beginning where the answers and the knowledge have been all along: within me.

To be a true master, the physical or external practice will not be enough. For the martial arts to be a true vehicle of training for the body, mind and spirit – and to survive the rapid escalation of sport-oriented martial arts – you need to forget about winning, being the best and being the strongest. Instead, you need to go within where you will be confronted with your strongest and most difficult opponent – yourself. Only then will your martial arts take on a far more profound meaning. And you will be on your way to truly becoming a master of life.

I don't think many people are ready to take on the inner martial arts journey. And it is not for the faint-hearted. Mankind is too comfortable with its misery, and would rather kill and destroy in the name of their religion than take the gracious act of becoming present and seeing that their thinking is the cause of their suffering. To train in the art of killing and expect people to live peacefully is a contradiction I am still studying.

It is within the nature of mankind to destroy on a whim, and to teach that martial arts will make you peaceful will only work for a very small minority. Even if the teachings are tempered with peaceful anecdotes, it is the mind's nature to exist and be recognised. And the martial arts give the ordinary person a perfect forum for this.

But all is not lost.

Become aware of the space between you and others. An awareness of that space means you can control it. Once you know about this space, you instantly become aware of how you move in others' space.

The missing link

Over the past 15 years I have continued my martial arts journey. With the influence of meditation, my teaching style has evolved and integrated what I consider to be the missing link in martial arts. For the first time, I have taken the influence of two great ju jitsu systems (Tenjin Shin-yo Ryu, one of the influences on modern judo, and Daito Ryu Aiki ju jitsu, the main influence on modern day Aikido), added the skills I have attained from taekwondo, Thai boxing, judo and wrestling, and seamlessly integrated mindful awareness and fitness to make it a real workout of body, mind and spirit.

I call this Northstar Ju Jitsu. This is the style of class I spent years looking for but never found. By embracing this methodology, the student is taught a way to learn the deadly moves of martial arts with an attitude of present awareness. This gives the student a mental space to choose to engage in conflict or not. This is truly the missing link that has been lost from martial arts in the race to update, evolve, win and above all else commercialise.

It has been my life's work so far to finally be able to understand what was missing from martial arts and then, by retaining certain traditional and cultural elements, use all of my experience to develop a style of martial arts that could be called a true workout for the body, mind and spirit, working from the inside out.

The beauty of this method of teaching is that the philosophy can easily be overlapped into daily life whereby you have the emotional space to choose peace in every interaction, truly becoming your own master in life.

Over the past 15 years Northstar Ju Jitsu has taught more than 10,000 students in ten locations, and now has an extensive online academy that opens up the opportunity for people all over the world to study Northstar Ju Jitsu.

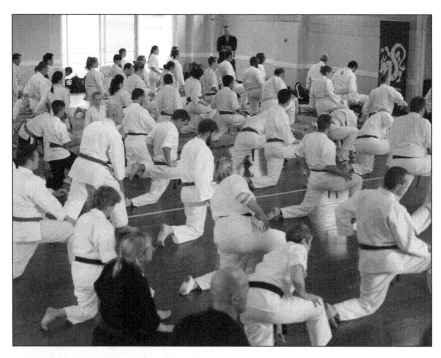

Northstar Ju Jitsu group class.

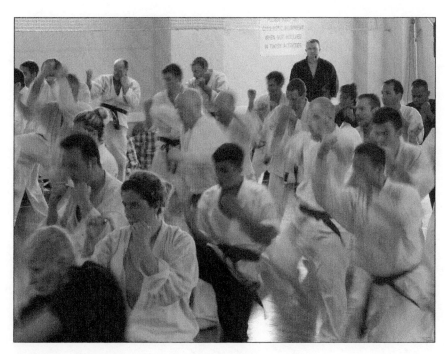

Watching over the students from the back of the class.

Chapter 12
My manifesto

I used to be incredibly goal driven. It served me well, and pushed me beyond my comfort zone. I adhered to the philosophy of top motivators and their advice on being the best you can be by having clearly defined goals for the days, months and years ahead. I used to worry if I did not have my weekly goals set out so they aligned with, and got me closer to, my ultimate goals. But I did achieve many goals over the years, and most involved dedication and endurance. None came easy.

But some goals are just not meant to be. And no matter how hard we try, life may just have other plans for us. Over the past 10 years, through the practice of meditation, I have felt a deeper connection with life. Instead of trying to force myself and my will on how I think life should be, I have come to realise that when you allow life to flow through you there is far less resistance to accepting the many daily dramas that colour our day. And in that awareness there is peace.

As part of this process, I have given up setting detailed goals. I do put 'out there' things I would like to happen, and I usually write them down but without a plan or time limit. Then I do something incredible, the opposite of what I used to do. I let life flow through me by not getting in its way, and let the goal or aspiration that is right for me manifest.

Since I started living my life this way I have married my soulmate, have an awesome relationship with my son, and live a powerful and productive life empowering others that in turn looks after my family finances. I am debt free.

But above everything I follow a calm meditative life in line with my choices of the heart. I feel truly blessed, and happy that I am exactly where I should be in life.

My new sparring partner

When I was first diagnosed with Parkinson's disease I got some great advice from Clyde Campbell, founder and CEO of the Shake It Up Foundation in Australia, who also has Parkinson's. He said, 'This is not the end of the journey. It is the beginning of a new journey to live each day being the best you can be, and to live life to the fullest by recognising, adjusting and doing whatever you can to live a positive and useful life that makes a difference'.

I never got caught up in 'Why me?' I can see the irony in working so hard to be incredibly fit for so many years and thinking my body is the centre of my universe, only to have it gradually lose function. I chose to take this as another experience on the journey of life that I can learn and grow from.

Ultimately, we all give up the body. It is just that the process for me has started sooner than I would have liked. But accepting deeply that it is part of life makes every day so much sweeter.

I don't want to sugarcoat this though. Parkinson's disease is not a walk in the park. It is a chronic and progressive neurological disease that affects millions of people worldwide. Though there is extensive worldwide research, and many new therapies are being developed, there is still no cure.

Just before I finish, I thought I would give you an insight into what my day looks like.

The earliest I will get up is 7am. I have tried earlier, but 7am fits me like a glove. Most mornings when I wake up, I leave behind the most

amazing, disturbing and totally illogical dreams. They have had me
singing, screaming, and kicking out fighting for my life. Poor Liz, my
wife. Sometimes I feel she is in my corner in a prize fight, as she gently
nudges me awake during the night to release me from this inner world.
I understand from my specialist, the brilliant Professor Rowe, that this is
called REM sleep disorder, and is one of the symptoms of Parkinson's you
do not hear about.

As I wake I am welcomed every morning by the tremor in my left arm.
This does not scare me or freak me out. Liz and I welcome it. We share
the experience by not trying to deny it or pretend it is not there. I used to
go from the bedroom to the meditation cushion, but these days Liz and I
enjoy a cuppa, waking up completely before I Zen out. Liz then prepares a
large glass of lemon juice in warm water and a glass of apple cider vinegar
for me to drink upon rising.

Before I meditate, I take my first round of meds – three capsules of Cu-
ATSM, which are part of a trial to see if we can slow down the progression.
I have not grown another leg or suffered any other side effects. I also take
my morning Sinamet, the main Parkinson's drug that masks most of the
symptoms. All set.

Then I head to the meditation cushion for 30 minutes, where I focus on
the breath, recite mantras, and sharpen my awareness. For so long the
meditation just seemed like a folly of half-sleep and light dreaming in
between moments of complete stillness. But I kept on. *The Bhagavad Gita*,
the famous Hindu spiritual masterpiece, has a great paragraph that I often
remind myself of: *'On this path, endeavour is never wasted, nor can it be repressed.
Even a very little practice protects one from great danger.'* It means that even if you
think the meditation is not working, behind the scenes it is actually making
a difference. During the 30 minutes – depending on the level of activity
going on in my head – the tremor will subside completely, and as I go into
the next part of my morning it will generally remain that way.

Getting up from the cushion, I used to make my way out to my own
personal dojo at the back of my house to stretch and continue my morning
practice. But these days my beautiful dojo is being used as a Pilates studio
so Liz can teach and we can both do reformer work from home. So now I

use the space in our large living/dining room area that looks directly out over our rear deck and Japanese gardens.

First up I do a very light stretch. Then I do a warm-up sequence taken from the 18 Lohan Chi Gong sequence. I have been studying Chi Gong for more than five years with Grand Master John Saw, taking private lessons at his home. Chi Gong is a set of stretches, movements, massage, breathing and meditation that moves and aligns the chi around the body. At best working to release blocked chi, it leads to a stronger healthier body. Most days I do my own yoga sequence that I have put together from various yoga schools. I intermix it with Chi Gong and Pilates, it takes 30 minutes at the most, and it maintains and improves my strength, flexibility and balance. It is quite vigorous, so it also warms me up and gets me puffing.

I love my pushbike. I ride every morning. Lately I have been doing a short sprint on the bike along the quiet waterfront a short ride from my home. I really push hard to a small park at the far end of the walkway, park my bike, and sit and listen to the morning sounds while reminding myself of how lucky I am to be able to sit in nature every morning. At the park I choose a short practice that may include fast walking up a grass hill a couple of times, one of the Chi Gong forms, or practice a part of my Tai Chi. Then I push my heart rate to the max as I do short sprints on the bike to get home, the entire ride taking me about 30 minutes.

Once home I generally go through some of my martial arts routines. They are fast and dynamic, and work speed, coordination and explosive movement. The entire process will take me anywhere from 60 to 120 minutes depending on other morning commitments.

You are probably wondering how I can do so much with the Parkinson's disease shadowing me. As you have already read, I have exercised most of my life. And like I have said, when the mind starts complaining or throwing up thoughts that are negative, I just ignore them and keep moving. Now I work within my limitations, be it age, injury or Parkinson's, and I just keep moving.

While cooling down I flick through Japanese language flash cards for ten minutes, revising words and vocabulary. I still continue to study Japanese, and attend a private lesson to sharpen my skills once per week.

Most days I fast from dinner the night before until 12pm. If I am not fasting, I generally eat a bowl of high-fibre muesli with psyllium husks, blueberries and natural yoghurt. I also really enjoy two hard-boiled eggs and Vegemite on sourdough twice per week. The number one must have for me every day is a homemade green smoothie. Fresh leafy greens, a Lebanese cucumber, and a kiwi fruit go into the blender ready to drink. I follow this up with a mixture of high-dose vitamin powder and vitamineral greens taken with vitamin D capsules, fish oil, a probiotic and milk thistle. That might sound like a lot, but I am literally supercharging myself and giving myself the best chance at maintaining a healthy immune system.

I finish my morning by reading a couple of pages from *The Gita*, a classical Hindu spiritual text. I also read from the modern spiritual classic, *I Am That* by Sri Nisargadatta Maharaj. They help me to keep it all in perspective.

I love my morning. There is now ample evidence in Parkinson's research that suggests exercise can reduce the symptoms. I feel that exercise that gets you puffing, no matter what it is, will improve general wellbeing and overall health. The softer exercises like Pilates, yoga, Chi Gong and Tai chi, will improve your flexibility, core strength and balance. The bottom line is, if you don't use it you will lose it. My entire morning routine helps me prepare for the Saturday sparring session with my top black belts.

I make my way into the small office beside my beautiful studio in Balmain. Running the martial arts schools, there is always something that needs attending to. I am lucky that Liz basically runs the office. I organise events and programs, and write blog posts. I also keep the online academy going smoothly.

At about 12pm I can usually start to feel the first round of Sinimet begin to wear off. My left hand starts to stiffen, making typing difficult, and I start to feel fatigue creep up on me. The tremor introduces itself again with a staccato of rapid movement on my left hand.

I take my second Sinimet at 12pm, and eat lunch while I wait for the medicine to kick in. I enjoy a simple lunch of salad and chicken or tuna. I try not to eat too much as I think in the West we all tend to overeat. I also stopped eating all sugars including sweets, chocolate, cakes and soft drinks years ago.

The fatigue lingers, so at about 1.30pm I go into my studio, lock the door and close the blinds, and do a 30-minute meditation and relaxation exercise called Yoga Nidra. I use the guided version by Swami Shankadev Saraswati. He has a great website called bigshakti.com. After 30 minutes I am suitably refreshed and ready to go into the rest of the day.

From 3.30pm onwards the first teaching team will arrive at the studio. They are a specialist group of kids trainers who excel in teaching the kids version of Northstar Ju Jitsu to various classes starting at three years old up to 16 years old. I do not teach the children's martial arts, although I spend a lot of time writing programs and training the trainers. From fourish I start to feel heavy and a little slow. It is hard to explain. My body feels like it is being weighed down by a thick wet blanket. No-one would know it because I just push through. But it takes all my strength to not go home and curl up on the couch.

At 5pm I take the last tablet for the day. This kicks in between 5pm and 6pm – just in time to sign in the adults for the 6.30pm class. By then, I am pretty much back to as close to normal as can be expected.

I do not teach the evening classes any more. Not because of the Parkinson's, but because I have an awesome team of adult Northstar Ju Jitsu instructors who do a great job of disseminating my teaching. I teach on Saturday mornings to mainly black belts, and run events such as seminars, gradings and the odd competition every couple of weeks.

As I mentioned, I still like to spar my top black belts on Saturday morning. I enjoy the challenge of holding my own and being able to be competitive. I move freely, and my techniques are still fast and on point. I think I will continue to spar for as long as I can.

You have to keep fighting. Even when the body is screaming at you to stop, just go one more round. In this way, Parkinson's does not tell me how to live. I choose to live first, then see if the Parkinson's will keep up.

After the evening class commences I head home. By the time I get home it is 7pm, and I have done my best with what I have today. Tomorrow may be different, but I will worry about that tomorrow. Liz and I share dinner, usually fish or chicken and variations of a raw Greek salad. Oh, and we enjoy a glass of red wine or two. A great end to a great day.

Parkinson's is not just a disease that affects the elderly. It does not discriminate, and many people like me in their early 50s are diagnosed every day. I could quite easily just give in and allow myself to fall into a pit of self-pity. But I am a fighter – always have been, always will be. So although I get self-conscious because I shake a little or my speech is slurred, I am determined to treat this like any other sparring partner – respect it, understand it, and know that if I let it, it could take me down. It is my intention to stay in the best shape possible physically, mentally and spiritually so that I will always be one step ahead of it.

At the same time, I continue to be a force to be reckoned with as I continue to study and pass on whatever I learn for as long as I can.

Teaching used to be easy for me. Now, teaching and motivating people has its challenges. But I intend to continue my journey and enjoy contributing to the lives of others. At the same time, I want to live my life to the fullest. It's going to have obstacles and challenges, but I've always been a fighter.

I may not fight the same way anymore, and I may now have new opponents. But I hope to be a role model to others who are affected by Parkinson's. I want to continue raising awareness about it, and to look to those who aim to slow its progression and find a cure.

When facing your own challenges, these are always going to be your biggest lessons. Because if you face them head on, regardless of the outcome, you're always going to stand tall. And that may be the biggest victory of all.

The End

Your next step

I invite you to connect with me and my community by joining my personal email list, Facebook and Instagram page, where I share everything from martial arts to health and fitness, meditation and spirituality, and how it has shaped my life and also helped my Parkinson's journey.

Just send an email to join my list.

Email: andy@nsma.com.au
Instagram: andydickinson
facebook.com/Northstarjujitsu
andydickinson.com.au
northstarmartialarts.com.au

Acknowledgements

A huge thank you to Valerie Khoo, you made this book happen. Bill Harper for your fine finishing touches on the manuscript. Linda Diggle for your expertise and guidance in making this a reality. My brother Robin, for your ongoing unconditional support. My brother John, who understands more than anyone else what it took and guided me through many ups and downs on this journey. May-lai, Darren, Mel, Matt, Jocelyn, Maree, Angus, Max, Rick, Ersel, Deb and Sophy and the entire kids team at Northstar for your support and dedication while I took time out to write the book. The league of strong men who I have learned so much and who always have my back including Vaughan Webster, Ed White, James Sassen, Steve Weston, Scott Brown, Phil Hinshelwood, Gordon Gilkes, Joe Bracks, Jebraun (Jimmy) Taouk, Joseph Williams, Chris Williams, Ernie Boggs, Alex Kostic and Dave Nowland. Clyde Campbell from the Shake It Up Foundation, an inspiration who is making a huge difference. Daryl Balkan, I have never forgotten your kindness and help when I was an unemployed fourth-year apprentice plumber. Tom, for being a constant shining example of patience, kindness and love between a father and son. Sifu John Saw and Sifu Alison Anderson, for your patience with me as I learn the softer arts. Dr Swami Shankardev Saraswati, for your patient guidance over the years. A huge thank you to Jay Laga'aia, Peter FitzSimons, Tom Cronin and Mark Dapin for your kind and sincere words. To all my training partners, sparring partners and competition opponents over the years who have all been instrumental in guiding me along the way, you helped me write this book.

Lastly, over the years I have been lucky enough to maintain a close relationship with my dad. Thanks Dad for being there for me when I really needed you. Blessed that I can share this book with you in the spirit of love and forgiveness.

About the Author

Andy is the founder and head of Northstar Ju Jitsu (NSJJ). He has spent more than 38 years training, competing and researching all aspects of martial arts and personal wellbeing worldwide. He is passionate about teaching martial arts as a legitimate path to understanding oneself and helping his students to see the link between training in the dojo and living a courageous life.

Andy has established a network of like-minded senior students who have gone on to teach Northstar Ju Jitsu within their own dojos, making NSJJ accessible throughout Sydney and Perth. He has also written and recorded a thorough online NSJJ Academy that adds a new dimension to the quality of how martial arts is taught and allows Northstar Ju Jitsu to be studied anywhere in the world.

An author of several eBooks and a prolific blogger, Andy presents education on a multitude of topics related to martial arts and life. Above all, Andy finds his greatest inspiration teaching all levels of students at his beautiful dojo in the heart of Sydney's inner west. His method of teaching is fun and he inspires the students to do their best by motivating them in a positive way at all times.